Gastroenteropancreatic System and Its Tumors: Part 1

Guest Editor

AARON I. VINIK, MD, PhD

ENDOCRINOLOGY AND METABOLISM CLINICS OF NORTH AMERICA

www.endo.theclinics.com

Consulting Editor
DEREK LEROITH, MD, PhD

December 2010 • Volume 39 • Number 4

SAUNDERS an imprint of ELSEVIER, Inc.

W.B. SAUNDERS COMPANY
A Division of Elsevier Inc.

1600 John F. Kennedy Boulevard • Suite 1800 • Philadelphia, Pennsylvania 19103-2899

http://www.theclinics.com

ENDOCRINOLOGY AND METABOLISM CLINICS OF NORTH AMERICA Volume 39, Number 4
December 2010 ISSN 0889-8529, ISBN-13: 978-1-4377-2447-9

Editor: Rachel Glover
Developmental Editor: Donald Mumford

Endocrinology and Metabolism Clinics of North America (ISSN 0889-8529) is published quarterly by Elsevier Inc., 360 Park Avenue South, New York, NY 10010-1710. Months of issue are March, June, September, and December. Periodicals postage paid at New York, NY and additional mailing offices. Subscription prices are USD 290.00 per year for US individuals, USD 503.00 per year for US institutions, USD 146.00 per year for US students and residents, USD 364.00 per year for Canadian individuals, USD 616.00 per year for Canadian institutions, USD 422.00 per year for international individuals, USD 616.00 per year for international institutions, and USD 216.00 per year for international and Canadian and foreign students/residents. To receive student/resident rate, orders must be accompanied by name of affiliated institution, date of term, and the signature of program/residency coordinator on institution letterhead. Orders will be billed at individual rate until proof of status is received. Foreign air speed delivery is included in all *Clinics* subscription prices. All prices are subject to change without notice. **POSTMASTER:** Send address changes to *Endocrinology and Metabolism Clinics of North America*, Elsevier Health Sciences Division, Subscription Customer Service, 3251 Riverport Lane, Maryland Heights, MO 63043. **Customer Service: Telephone: 1-800-654-2452** (U.S. and Canada); **1-314-447-8871** (outside U.S. and Canada). **Fax: 1-314-447-8029. E-mail: journalscustomerservice-usa@elsevier.com** (for print support); **journalsonlinesupport-usa@elsevier.com** (for online support).

Reprints. For copies of 100 or more, of articles in this publication, please contact the Commercial Rights Department, Elsevier Inc., 360 Park Avenue South, New York, NY 10010-1710; phone: (+1) 212-633-3813; fax: (+1) 212-462-1935; e-mail: reprints@elsevier.com.

Endocrinology and Metabolism Clinics of North America is covered in *MEDLINE/PubMed (Index Medicus)*, *EMBASE/Excerpta Medica*, *Current Contents/Clinical Medicine*, *Current Contents/Life Sciences*, *Science Citation Index*, *ISI/BIOMED*, *BIOSIS*, and *Chemical Abstracts*.

Printed and bound by CPI Group (UK) Ltd, Croydon, CR0 4YY

Transferred to Digital Print 2011

Contributors

CONSULTING EDITOR

DEREK LEROITH, MD, PhD
Chief, Division of Endocrinology, Metabolism, and Bone Diseases, Department
of Medicine, Mount Sinai School of Medicine, New York, New York

GUEST EDITOR

AARON I. VINIK, MD, PhD, FCP, MACP
Research Director of Strelitz Diabetes Center and Director of the Neuroendocrine Unit,
EVMS Strelitz Diabetes Research Center, Eastern Virginia Medical School,
Norfolk, Virginia

AUTHORS

CATHERINE T. ANTHONY, PhD
Senior Postdoctoral Researcher, Department of Surgery, Louisiana State University
Health Sciences Center, New Orleans, Louisiana

JOY E.S. ARDILL, PhD, MRCPath
Professor of Medicine, Queen's University; Consultant Clinical Scientist, Regional
Regulatory Peptide Laboratory, Royal Victoria Hospital, Belfast, United Kingdom

STEPHEN R. BLOOM, MA, MD, DSc, FRCPath, FRCP, FMedSci
Professor, Section of Investigative Medicine, Imperial College London, London,
United Kingdom

LEIGH ANNE KAMERMAN BURNS, MS, LDN, RD
Instructor of Clinical Medicine/Nutrition, Cancer Prevention Liaisons, Louisiana State
University Health Sciences Center, School of Medicine New Orleans, Stanley S. Scott
Cancer Center, New Orleans, Louisiana

JESSICA CHANG, BND, MBBS
Clinical Research Fellow, Discipline of Medicine, Royal Adelaide Hospital, University
of Adelaide; Centre of Clinical Research Excellence in Nutritional Physiology,
Interventions, and Outcomes, Adelaide, South Australia, Australia

HERBERT CHEN, MD, FACS
Professor and Vice-Chairman, Department of Surgery, University of Wisconsin Carbone
Cancer Center, Madison, Wisconsin

EMANUEL CHRIST, MD, PhD
Division of Endocrinology, Diabetology, and Clinical Nutrition, University Hospital
of Berne Inselspital, Berne, Switzerland

CHANTAL DREYER, MD
Department of Medical Oncology, Beaujon University Hospital (AP-HP, Paris 7 Diderot), Clichy, France

SANDRINE FAIVRE, MD, PhD
Department of Medical Oncology, Beaujon University Hospital (APHP, Paris 7 Diderot), Clichy, France

VAY LIANG W. GO, MD
Distinguished Professor of Medicine and Director, UCLA Center for Excellence in Pancreatic Diseases, David Geffen School of Medicine at UCLA, Los Angeles, California

MICHAEL HOROWITZ, MBBS, PhD
Professor, Discipline of Medicine, Royal Adelaide Hospital, University of Adelaide; Centre of Clinical Research Excellence in Nutritional Physiology, Interventions, and Outcomes, Adelaide, South Australia, Australia

FREDIANO INZANI, MD
Institute of Anatomic Pathology, Universitá Cattolica del Sacro Cuore—Policlinico A. Gemelli, Rome; Department of Human Pathology and Heredity, University of Pavia, Pavia, Italy

KAREN L. JONES, PhD
Associate Professor, Discipline of Medicine, Royal Adelaide Hospital, University of Adelaide; Centre of Clinical Research Excellence in Nutritional Physiology, Interventions, and Outcomes, Adelaide, South Australia, Australia

ERIC H. LIU, MD
Associate Professor, Division of Surgical Oncology and Endocrine Surgery, Vanderbilt University, Medical Center, Nashville, Tennessee

JOHN LYONS III, MD
Chief Surgical Resident, Department of Surgery, Louisiana State University Health Sciences Center, New Orleans, Louisiana

KJELL OBERG, MD, PhD
Professor, Department of Endocrine Oncology, University Hospital, Uppsala, Sweden

THOMAS M. O'DORISIO, MD
Professor, Department of Internal Medicine, Division of Endocrinology/Metabolism/Diabetes, University of Iowa Hospitals and Clinics, Iowa City, Iowa

GARY L. PITTENGER, PhD
Associate Professor and Director, Protein Chemistry, Departments of Internal Medicine and Anatomy and Pathology, Strelitz Diabetes Center, Norfolk, Virginia

ERIC RAYMOND, MD, PhD
Department of Medical Oncology, Beaujon University Hospital (AP-HP, Paris 7 Diderot), Clichy, France

CHRISTOPHER K. RAYNER, MBBS, PhD
Associate Professor, Discipline of Medicine, Royal Adelaide Hospital, University of Adelaide; Centre of Clinical Research Excellence in Nutritional Physiology, Interventions, and Outcomes, Adelaide, South Australia, Australia

JEAN CLAUDE REUBI, MD
Division of Cell Biology and Experimental Cancer Research, Institute of Pathology, University of Berne, Berne, Switzerland

GUIDO RINDI, MD, PhD
Institute of Anatomic Pathology, Università Cattolica del Sacro Cuore—Policlinico A. Gemelli, Rome, Italy

MARIE-PAULE SABLIN, MD
Department of Medical Oncology, Beaujon University Hospital (AP-HP, Paris 7 Diderot), Clichy, France

KATHERINE A. SIMPSON, MB, ChB, MRCP
Section of Investigative Medicine, Imperial College London, London, United Kingdom

ENRICO SOLCIA, MD
Department of Human Pathology and Heredity, University of Pavia, Pavia, Italy

PRIYA SRIHARI
UCLA Center for Excellence in Pancreatic Diseases, David Geffen School of Medicine at UCLA, Los Angeles, California

DAVID A. TAYLOR-FISHWICK, PhD
Associate Professor and Director, Cell, Molecular and Islet Biology, Departments of Internal Medicine and Microbiology and Molecular Cell Biology, Strelitz Diabetes Center, Norfolk, Virginia

DAMIAN WILD, MD
Department of Nuclear Medicine, University Hospital Freiburg, Freiburg, Germany; Institute of Nuclear Medicine, University College London, London, United Kingdom

EUGENE A. WOLTERING, MD, FACS
Section Chief of Surgical Oncology and Endocrine Surgery; The James D. Rives Professor of Surgery and Neuroscience; Director of Surgical Research, Department of Surgery, Louisiana State University Health Sciences Center, New Orleans, Louisiana

BARBARA ZAREBCZAN, MD
Endocrine Surgery Research Laboratories, Department of Surgery, University of Wisconsin Carbone Cancer Center, Wisconsin Institutes for Medical Research, Madison, Wisconsin

Contents

energy need. Gut hormones are released after a meal and signal to the brain to initiate meal termination and feelings of satiation. However, reward pathways are able to override this mechanism so that when palatable food is presented, food is consumed irrespective of energy requirements.

a GLP-1 analog that has a longer half-life than GLP-1. Targeting GLP-1R by ^{111}In-DOTA-exendin-4 or ^{111}In-DPTA-exendin-4 offers a new approach that permits the successful localization of small benign insulinomas. It is likely that this new noninvasive technique has the potential to replace the invasive localization by selective arterial stimulation and venous sampling.

Barbara Zarebczan and Herbert Chen

Although neuroendocrine tumors are rare, the more common types such as gastrointestinal and pancreatic carcinoids, medullary thyroid cancers, and small cell lung cancers have been studied in detail during the last few years. Data published thus far indicate that multiple signaling pathways are involved in these cancers. Recent focus has been on developing novel therapeutics by targeting specific signaling pathways. This article details several of the signaling mechanisms that have been discovered to play a role in the development and progression of neuroendocrine tumors. The therapeutic options developed to address the various pathways, including their specific mechanisms of actions, are also discussed.

Sandrine Faivre, Marie-Paule Sablin, Chantal Dreyer, and Eric Raymond

Neuroendocrine tumors (NETs) are rare malignancies that arise from endocrine cells located in various anatomic locations, with a dramatic increase in incidence during the last 30 years. Limited therapeutic options are currently available for patients with advanced well-differentiated NETs, including carcinoids and pancreatic NETs. Streptozotocin-based chemotherapy and somatostatin analogues are drugs that are currently used for the treatment of progressive metastatic NETs. Recently, sunitinib demonstrating efficacy in pancreatic islet cell carcinomas has opened a new avenue for the treatment of NETs, and further trials shall be considered in NET types such as carcinoids, poorly differentiated neuroendocrine carcinomas, and several other endocrine tumors that depend on vascular endothelial growth factor (VEGF)/VEGF receptor for angiogenesis. In addition, drugs with distinct mechanisms of action, such as mammalian target of rapamycin inhibitors, currently investigated in phase 3 trials, may also supply novel options to control tumor growth and metastasis. Although acknowledged as rare tumors, recent data demonstrated the feasibility of large randomized trials in this disease. Furthermore, data from large trials also showed the importance of selecting an appropriate patient population when designing randomized studies. This review focuses on novel therapeutic approaches in the treatment of well-differentiated NETs. Based on recent data, novel strategies may now be designed using those anticancer agents to optimize the current treatment of patients with NETs.

Vay Liang W. Go, Priya Srihari, and Leigh Anne Kamerman Burns

Gastroenteropancreatic (GEP) neuroendocrine tumors (NETs) are relatively rare neoplasms that characteristically synthesize and secrete an

THE CLINICS ARE NOW AVAILABLE ONLINE!

Access your subscription at:
www.theclinics.com

Foreword

Gastroenteropancreatic System and Its Tumors: Part 1

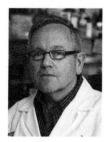

Derek LeRoith, MD, PhD
Consulting Editor

This is the first issue of two on the neuroendocrine system compiled by Dr Arthur (Aaron) Vinik, a world-renowned leader in this field. While most physicians only occasionally consider this system and the tumors that develop, I believe readers will be surprised how important the system is, both in understanding the normal physiology and pathology, and in how commonly disorders arise in our patients.

In a rather fascinating article, Drs Liu and Oberg describe the history of the gastroenteropancreatic (GEP) system. Major discoveries in relation to the structure, physiology, biochemistry, hormones, assays, and tumors in this system have been made over the past century, and many of those responsible for these discoveries have received Nobel prizes for their work. Undoubtedly these discoveries have formed the fundamentals of our understanding, not only of the GEP system, but also of many other physiologic and pathologic systems in the body. In 1902, Bayliss and Starling made the observation that nutrients instilled into the duodenum stimulate pancreatic exocrine secretion, and so arose the notion that a substance produced in one part of the body could excite a response in another (hormone = excite), leading to the discovery of the endocrine nature of the GEP system. Since that time, there have been discoveries of many hormones seeking functions, functions seeking a hormone, and physiologic and pathologic events yet to be linked to the GEP system. In these two issues many of the new and novel discoveries and applications of this science will be addressed.

Gastrointestinal neoplasms are often neuroendocrine in origin and may be nonfunctional or functional in respect to releasing bioactive amines or hormones. In their article, Drs Rindi, Inzani, and Solcia describe in detail the development and prognosis of these tumors that can occur throughout the gastrointestinal tract, in many instances arising from dysplastic or hyperplastic regions. In many instances the prognosis may be quite poor, despite attempts at therapeutic intervention that include surgery, radiation, and

Endocrinol Metab Clin N Am 39 (2010) xiii–xvi
doi:10.1016/j.ecl.2010.09.004
0889-8529/10/$ – see front matter © 2010 Elsevier Inc. All rights reserved.

endo.theclinics.com

chemotherapy. This is particularly true of tumors that have a high mitotic index and elevated Ki67 index of proliferation. There is a clear reduction in survival if diagnosed late at an advanced stage of the disease, dictating a better means of early recognition.

As discussed by Drs Simpson and Bloom, food intake is controlled by the hypothalamus and brain stem, and there are numerous hormonal inputs affecting appetite and satiety. Many of these emanate from the gastrointestinal (GI) tract, others, for example, from adipose tissue signals. Generally appetite can be controlled by these signals in relationship to energy requirements; however, apparently when "rewarding" types of food are ingested, there are mechanisms that can override the normal control mechanisms. The authors discuss how this overriding mechanism(s) may be a factor in the increasing incidence of overweight and obese individuals.

It has now become recognized that the stomach is the second major regulator of blood glucose levels after insulin, and new and emerging evidence suggests that there may be a transition in early diabetes from rapid gastric emptying to gastroparesis in longstanding diabetes, having major different consequences on blood glucose regulation, and of course the choices of therapy. In addition there is a brake mechanism in which the pancreas secretes hIAPP to slow the stomach emptying, thereby reducing postprandial hyperglycemia, which breaks down in diabetes, and the duodenum produces Ghrelin, which accelerates emptying.

Chang, Rayner, Jones, and Horowitz describe the underlying mechanisms involved in these processes. Cellular atrophy, neuropathy, and lack of NO production due to reduced expression of NO synthase in enteric cells all affect the process. Changes in the secretion of hormones, including Ghrelin, and hIAPP, among others, are implicated. Scintigraphy and stable isotope breath tests are among the many diagnostic tests available, although these two seem more useful than the others. Similarly, treatment regimes, while available, are limited in their usefulness, but new and promising therapies are being directed at the hormones involved such as Ghrelin agonists.

The gastrointestinal tract and the pancreatic ductal system are sites of residence of adult, protodifferentiated stem cells, which can be harnessed to develop into adult physiologically functioning cells. Drs Taylor-Fishwick and Pittenger discuss the possibility of using these stem cells to differentiate into islet cells for transplantation in diabetic patients. As described, while islet cell transplantation can be preferable over pancreatic transplantation due to lower morbidity, availability remains a major problem. Numerous studies have described the increased numbers of beta cells from ductal precursors, transdifferentiated from other cell types. In this article they focus on the possibility of regeneration from existing stem cells in the islets.

Neuroendocrine tumors of the GEP axis may be divided into NETs or pancreatic NETS, referred to as PNETs. Once considered relatively rare, the incidence has increased five-fold over the last two decades compared with a lack of increase of all other GI neoplasms. The prevalence of NETS is greater than all other pancreatic and GI neoplasms combined. Whether this relates to a real increase in incidence, or simply an enhanced awareness or better means of detection needs to be resolved. Neuroendocrine tumors are often difficult to diagnose and often delayed for many years, as Drs Ardill and Tom O'Dorisio describe in their article. This is often due to the tumors being asymptomatic, or the symptoms being vague and intermittent and often similar to symptoms associated with other conditions.

One of the gold standards for identifying these tumors is using appropriate biochemical markers combined with scintigraphic techniques, using radioactive somatostatin tracers that bind to the type 2 and 5 somatostatin receptor subtypes present in many NETs but relatively scarce in PNETs. However, these radiographic techniques are often unable to detect the small tumors and therefore biological markers have been successfully used such as Chromogranin A, which is used both as a diagnostic tool as well as a prognostic marker. A number of other biomarkers, classically those for phaechromocytomas or pancreastin, pancreatic polypeptide, and gastrin, are also useful. However, there is obviously a need for more specific markers to help in the diagnosis of these tumors.

Glucagon-like peptide-1 (GLP-1) and its analogues are currently used in the management of diabetes. The GLP-1 receptor (GLP-1R) is also widely expressed on different normal tissues and also on some tumors. Insulinomas express high levels, and as described in the article by Christ, Wild, and Reubi, newer radioactive isotope techniques are being developed using isotope-labeled chelated exendin-4 (an analogue of GLP-1) as the probe. Success with this technique could replace other techniques including arteriography and venous sampling in PNETs.

As discussed by Drs Zarebczan and Chen, there has been extensive investigation on neuroendocrine tumors and the signaling pathways that are involved in their development and progression, important targets for potential therapeutics. These pathways include the PI3K/Akt and MAPK pathways and their downstream effectors such as GSK3b and mTOR, as well as the Notch and RET signaling pathways. A number of inhibitors of these pathways are already in trials for various tumors, such as medullary carcinoma of the thyroid and the use of tyrosine kinase inhibitors.

In addition to standard therapies available for neuroendocrine tumors that are malignant and metastasize, Drs Faivre, Sablin, Dreyer, and Raymond describe some new options that are being tested. The standards of therapy of NETs include the use of somatostatin, which is second only to insulin as peptide therapy for endocrine and hormonal disorders. However, the control of symptoms remains their major target and little effects of standard chemotherapy have proven to be effective in NETs. More recently new and exciting data is emerging with the use of Tyrosine Kinase inhibitors as well as MTOR inhibitors for NETs which seem to be particularly effective in PNETs. An example is Sunitinib, an inhibitor of VEGF/VEGF receptor signaling that has a fairly strong effect on angiogenesis, and mTOR inhibitors have been shown to inhibit aggressive tumor that also metastasize. There is therefore hope that in the near future these and other drugs will be available for these severe situations.

In a separate article Drs Go, Srihari, and Burns deal with the nutrition support of the patients with these tumors. The importance of this topic relates to the neuroamines and hormones released by the tumors that affect both pancreatic exocrine and gastrointestinal function. Active substances may include VIP, gastrin, ghrelin, somatostatin, glucagon, and others that lead to these GI disturbances and loss of nutrients and minerals. Nutritional counseling and the value of the nutritionist are stressed in this article, as well as some practical references.

Angiogenesis, whereby new vessels are formed, often under the influence of VEGF and its receptors, plays an important role in tumor growth. Somatostatin analogues were found early on that have anti-angiogenic function and were thought to explain some of their effects on tumor growth, in addition to effects on inhibiting hormone secretion from endocrine tumors. In pursuing this concept, Drs Lyons, Anthony, and Woltering describe in vitro studies on other inhibitors of angiogenesis in human tumor tissues, leading to the use of some of these inhibitors in early human trials in carcinoids, for example, that have had some success.

Readers are reminded that another issue will be forthcoming covering other aspects of this important topic.

Derek LeRoith, MD, PhD
Division of Endocrinology, Metabolism, and Bone Diseases
Department of Medicine
Mount Sinai School of Medicine
One Gustave L. Levy Place
Box 1055, Altran 4-36
New York, NY 10029, USA

E-mail address:
derek.leroith@mssm.edu

Preface

Gastroenteropancreatic System and Its Tumors: Part 1

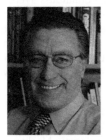

Aaron I. Vinik, MD, PhD, FCP, MACP
Guest Editor

Who would have thought that the simple act of instilling acid in the duodenum led to flow of juice from the denervated pancreas, which would lead to the discovery of the hormone secretin and the endocrine system, the first gastrointestinal hormone, and a whole new discipline, that of gastrointestinal neuroendocrinology? Who would have thought that the brain would talk to the gut and this would be a reciprocal relationship? As a scientist who has had his head buried in the GI endocrine system for decades (figuratively speaking), it has been a wonderful journey from the Cinderella discipline to front stage or close to it. In this issue of the *Endocrinology Clinics*, much of what has transpired in the evolution of this discipline is presented by world authorities who deserve special recognition for their contributions as well as the superiority of their science and their perseverance with the foster child. The discipline has led to several Nobel prizes as well as burying careers in dead ends with hormones that have yet to fulfill a function. There have also been surprises such as the discovery that the gut could tell the brain when it should restrict eating behavior even if many human brains ignore the signal. This area of endeavor is of particular importance with the explosion in worldwide obesity, and any material that could alter brain recalcitrance ought to have a place in changing human self-destructive behavior. In the world of diabetes we have come to recognize the role of insulin in regulating blood glucose, and more recently have rediscovered the important role that glucagon plays in preventing hypoglycemia, which itself is the leading cause of noncompliance with anti-diabetes medications and treatment failures. Little did we know that the stomach would turn out to be the second major regulator of blood glucose concentrations and that the mechanism for altering the rate of gastric emptying by gut hormones would be a central cause of brittle diabetes and possibly amenable to therapy with yet another gastrointestinal hormone. Of course, we have come to assume that the GI system always

Endocrinol Metab Clin N Am 39 (2010) xvii–xviii
doi:10.1016/j.ecl.2010.09.005
0889-8529/10/$ – see front matter © 2010 Elsevier Inc. All rights reserved.

behaves in an exemplary fashion, but just as with other tissues, unbridled growth and proliferation of the protodifferentiated cell can lead to tumor formation that creates interesting and challenging clinical syndromes, enough to tax the ingenuity of any and every specialty. This challenge has been admirably met by the discovery that GI hormone receptors and radiotracers can now be used to localize these tumors and even be embraced for peptide receptor radiotherapy for the tumor annihilation. Pathologists have now finally come to an agreement on what constitutes a reasonable staging that relates to prognosis, and surprisingly that well-differentiated tumors can be metastatic with an expectation of survival for years with appropriate management. Novel anticancer management with tyrosine kinase inhibitors and MTOR inhibitors have now found their way into the world of NETS and pathways beyond are being discovered. Now the slipper fits Cinderella, who has the glass slippers to wear to the ball.

Aaron I. Vinik, MD, PhD, FCP, MACP
EVMS Strelitz Diabetes Research Center
Eastern Virginia Medical School
855 West Brambleton Avenue
Norfolk, VA 23510-1001, USA

E-mail address:
vinikai@evms.edu

The History and Development of the Gastroenteropancreatic Endocrine Axis

Eric H. Liu, MD[a], Kjell Oberg, MD, PhD[b],*

KEYWORDS

- Gastroenteropancreatic endocrine axis • Hormones
- Secretin • Insulin • Somatostatin • Somatostatin analogs
- PRRT

The history of the gastroenteropancreatic (GEP) endocrine axis is a rich heritage filled with glorious stories of triumphant discoveries and miracle cures. However, it is also filled with drama, clash of egos and personalities, and reformulations of previous dogma. While scientists slowly developed new concepts of a diffuse neuroendocrine system, at the center of these stories were patients suffering from mysterious syndromes and childhood death. A few historic names in the field of medicine include Bayliss, Starling, Banting, Kocher, Whipple, and Cushing; their work has been honored by numerous Nobel prizes and immortalized in the medical language spoken by generations of physicians and scientists. Through their work, a mature concept of the endocrine system has emerged not only in the traditional secretory organs, but also in the vast and diffuse digestive system. Fundamental medical principles, such as hormone action, distant physiologic regulation, and ductless secretion were once mysteries. They now form the basis of basic medical diagnostics and therapeutics. This article discusses and reviews the rich history that served as the foundation of modern medicine, from the early descriptions of tumors, to the discovery of hormones and assays, and how they resulted in the treatments available today.

EARLY DESCRIPTIONS OF THE GEP ENDOCRINE AXIS

Ancient physicians recognized the importance of certain glands in disease. The Chinese described the role of the goiters in the thyroid, and the Egyptians saw the ovaries as crucial to female reproduction.[1,2] But it was not until Galen that the concept of vital spirits was developed in his studies of the pituitary in the second century.[3] The description of

[a] Department of Surgery, Surgical Oncology, Vanderbilt University, Medical Center, Nashville, TN, USA
[b] Department of Endocrine Oncology, University Hospital, SE-751 85 Uppsala, Sweden
* Corresponding author.
E-mail address: kjell.oberg@medsci.uu.se

Endocrinol Metab Clin N Am 39 (2010) 697–711
doi:10.1016/j.ecl.2010.09.002
0889-8529/10/$ – see front matter © 2010 Elsevier Inc. All rights reserved.

glands took on greater meaning over the centuries as anatomists examined both ductal and ductless organs, and secretions could find their way into other structures or directly into the blood. In 1907, Sir Edward Sharpey-Schäfer produced a model that unified the various glandular organs into one comprehensive physiologic system.[4]

The principle of endocrine regulation was originated by Claude Bernard based on the concepts of homeostasis.[5] He used the term internal secretion in his descriptions of the liver as an important component of homeostasis. These concepts matured quickly with the classical endocrine organs, such as the adrenals, the thyroid, and the lymphatics by the work of Thomas Addison, John Hunter, Theodor Kocher, and Charles Edouard Brown Sequard.[6–9] The descriptions of the GEP endocrine system were more complicated and required the new technology of microscopy before they could be investigated. Paul Langerhans as a medical student in 1869 then was able to describe small islands in the pancreas that would emerge as the islets of Langerhans, and Nikolai Kulchitsky described the clear cells in the crypts of Lieber-kühn that now bear his name.[10,11] While these were clearly important early discoveries, they were purely descriptive, as no function could be attributed to any of these cells. The concept of a chemical messenger would have to wait until the turn of the 20th century in one of the most famous experiments in medicine.

THE GUT AS AN ENDOCRINE ORGAN: SECRETIN

The dominant paradigm of gut physiology was the concept of nervism, developed first by Karl Ludwig, then solidified by Ivan Pavlov and his famous dogs.[12–14] That evidence stated that the nervous system was the regulator of bodily functions. In the specific case of digestive secretion, Leon Popielski and E. Wertheimer tested the role of nerves in the regulation of pancreatic secretion in response to duodenal acidification by aggressively denervating the abdominal organs in dogs and cats.[15] In all instances, they could not unlink the acid from the secretion, leading them both to conclude that dedicated reflex nerves existed exclusively between the duodenum and the pancreas. William Bayliss and Ernest Starling engaged the question of gastrointestinal secretion by repeating the denervation experiments by Popieslki and Wertheimer, but with a small modification.[16]

On Jan. 16, 1902, they concentrated the denervation to an isolated loop of jejunum, carefully skeletonizing the intestines such that only the mesenteric vessels remained.[17] Dilute hydrochloric acid was introduced into the bowel, and a steady flow of pancreatic juice resulted, exactly as occurred in the duodenum. This simple experiment showed that blood alone could carry a signal to start pancreatic secretion. As a follow-up, they created an extract from scraped jejunal mucosa and injected it intravenously, again causing a free flow of pancreatic fluid. They even showed that boiling did not destroy the effect, and it could not be duplicated from distal ileal tissue. At that moment, Starling declared, "Then it must be a chemical reflex." Confident with this discovery, they went on to present these data 6 days later at the Royal Society, calling their newly discovered agent secretin. Before its publication in September, other scientists were able to replicate these results and support grew for the chemical messenger theory.[18] In fact, Pavlov himself repeated the experiment in late 1902, stating, "Of course, they are right. It is clear that we did not take out an exclusive patent for the discovery of truth."[19] These experiments led to the eventual development of and coining of the word hormone (derived from the Greek "to excite") by William Hardy to describe chemical messengers as a class of physiologic regulators.[20] In the following years, Starling recognized that the gland secretion was in fact under dual control of both circulating chemicals and nerves. Thus was the birth of the GEP neuroendocrine system.

Other hormonal discoveries soon followed. Langley, Anderson, and Elliot were studying adrenaline; Dale described histamine in 1910, and Edkins described the potential existence of gastrin in 1905.[21–23] In the Croonian lecture to the Royal College of Physicians, Starling not only cited those works, but also addressed the potential of sex hormones and the antidiabetic effects of the pancreas.[20] The discovery of new GEP hormones would continue throughout the century and continues today. The doctrine of hormone regulation would provide the platform for further discoveries that not only influenced the understanding of the gut, but also the development of techniques broadly used throughout science and medicine.

THE MOST FAMOUS HORMONE OF ALL: INSULIN

The discovery of secretin was a discovery of the fundamental physiologic pathway in the GEP system. However, very few people died of secretin deficiency. Diabetes, however, was a disease with a 100% mortality, and in children, it was a diagnosis worse than cancer. Any new therapy would be accepted as an advance, but the discovery of insulin was much more: for most, it was truly a miracle cure.[24]

The underlying mechanism was not well understood, but the symptoms were well described. Since the Egyptians first recorded the sweet urine from diabetics, it was known to be a disorder of sugars. Patients all developed the classical symptoms of polydipsia, polyuria, fatigue, and frequently coma.[25–29] But there was no understanding of the different types of diabetes. No one understood the difference between what is now known as type 1 diabetes (autoimmune, or juvenile) versus type 2 diabetes (insulin resistance, or adult-onset).[30] The state-of-the-art therapy was championed by Dr Frederick M. Allen, the leading authority at the time. From his studies at Rockerfeller University in New York, he developed a treatment of Draconian calorie restriction.[31–33] He recommended that diabetics only consume as much food as they could metabolize. At the time that meant fasting until clearing of glucosuria. Then small amounts of food were given until tolerance levels were achieved, which sometimes meant only a few hundred calories a day. This left patients emaciated and lethargic, but could extend their lives for a few months. Until the discovery of insulin, there was no other option; prominent diabetologists, including Elliott Joslin of Boston, could only starve their patients until they were living skeletons.[34] Allen opened a clinic in New Jersey, and the most prominent Americans went to him for treatment. It was understood, however, that once the symptoms set in, that death was not far, especially in children.

A young Canadian, army surgeon with farming roots, Frederick Banting, would find himself at the Univeristy of Toronto, not because of his brilliance, but more because his private practice was slow to establish.[35] He took a lecturing position at the university to supplement his income. In the fall of 1920, while preparing for a student lecture on the pancreas, Banting noted that the islets of Langerhans are preserved in gallstone pancreatitis, inspiring a short entry in his notebook:

"Diabetes, ligate pancreatic ducts of dogs. Keep dogs alive till acini degenerate leaving Islets. Try to isolate the internal secretion of these to relieve glycosuria."

In May 1921, Banting, working with Professor J.J.R. Macleod, and a young medical student, Charles Best, began work on the project. The experiment was straight forward; Banting would open the abdomen of a dog, locate and ligate the pancreatic duct, close the animal, and allow the exocrine tissue to die away. Several weeks later, he would go back into the abdomen, perform a total pancreatectomy on the atrophied gland and either graft it into another pancreatectomized dog, or try to develop an extract of the internal secretion. Initially, it was Macleod who taught Banting how to perform the two-stage procedure. The standard method was to perform a near-total pancreatectomy that did not cause diabetes. The pancreatic remnant was sutured subcutaneously and the animal allowed to recover (note that the pancreas in a dog is more diffuse than a human gland, which has a firm shape). In the second stage, the remaining pancreas was removed, and the animal quickly became diabetic, usually dying within a week. After establishing this technique, Banting went on to the duct ligation. In a healthy animal, this procedure proved difficult; the duct was small and hard to find, and it was easy to ligate pancreatic tissue instead of the duct.

Banting and Best used their allotted animals faster than they anticipated, but they were able to procure stray dogs for their experiments, a common practice of the time. Meanwhile, Macleod had left the university for summer vacation in Scotland. It was a hot summer of work. The laboratories were hot, and the operating facilities smelled of animal flesh. When they operated, their animals kept dying of infections, because they could not keep the sweat or flies from entering the surgical field. When the dogs were able to survive, they did not produce the desired results. When Banting went in to recover the atrophied organ, he found a perfectly normal one. Several animals were religated; several died in the process. Eventually a few dogs did atrophy, and their organs were ground up and a liquid extraction prepared. They gave the extract to a diabetic depancreatized dog, and it lowered its blood sugars. Later experiments would wake dogs from diabetic comas and dramatically lower blood sugar levels.[36] Further tests with extract from fetal cow, then adult cow pancreas would continue to be successful, leading to the refinement of extract with the help of a new colleague, J.B. Collip. They called this extract, isletin, which would later be known as insulin.[37] Unfortunately, as experiments succeeded, relationships failed. The country boy, Banting, saw the intellectual professor, MacLeod, as stealing the credit. He saw Collip as taking over by producing better extract. In the beginning of 1922, at the first human test, Leonard Thompson, a charity care boy with diabetes, down to 65 pounds, was given a crude extract prepared by Banting and Best. It failed to lower his blood glucose. The failure was crushing to Banting. Two weeks later, however, after Collip had optimized the extraction process, another dose was given to Thompson; this time the results were truly spectacular. The boy's blood sugar dropped; his ketouria resolved, and he revived from a near comatose state. Patients from all over North America descended upon Toronto. While this stunning success should have led to celebration, it destroyed the dynamic of the team, and paranoia set in. Eventually, Banting and Best received recognition for their early work; Banting and MacLeod shared the Nobel Prize for Medicine in 1923.

The miracle of insulin itself as a cure for deadly disease is enough drama alone, but later in the century, insulin would find itself at the center of another race, to produce the first recombinant hormone medication. It gave birth to huge pharmaceutical companies such as Eli Lily, Novo Nordic, and Genentech.[38] It provided Nobel prizes to Frederick Sanger in 1958 (it was the first protein ever sequenced), Dorothy Crowfoot Hodgkin in 1969 (it was the first protein whose structure was determined by radiographic crystallography), and Rosalyn Sussman Yalow in 1977 (who developed the first radioimmunoassay [RIA]against insulin).[39–43]

TUMORS OF THE GEP: CARCINOID

Classical carcinomas of the small bowel were rare entities, but they had characteristic pathologic features.[44] However, a small series of patients with ileal tumors defied this typical pathologic diagnosis. In 1867, Theodor Langhans first described a small, firm, mushroom-shaped submucosal tumor from a 50-year-old woman who died of tuberculosis.[45] He noted the unusual fact that it had sharp borders without any evidence of peritumoral invasion, with nests of rich, thick fibrous stroma. Twenty-one years later, another series of patients was described by Otto Lubarsch, where ileal tumors were found with tubercular growth patterns.[46] He did note that diarrhea had been a prominent symptom in one of the patients, consistent with the modern understanding of these tumors. In Lubarsch's review of the literature, he recognized that these tumors were not consistent with carcinomas. Soon after, William Ransom described a case of a 50-year-old woman with the symptoms of menorrhagia, abdominal masses, and severe diarrhea with wheezing.[47] At the time, her symptoms were attributed to uterine fibroids, but on autopsy, she was found to have several ileal nodules and hepatic tumors. He noted that there was some malignant potential and termed them "glandular carcinomas."

The description of these tumors that has endured to modern times is attributed to Siegfried Oberndorfer in 1907.[48] His seminal paper first introduced the term karzinoide to describe a series of patients with unusual tumors. His first case also involved a patient who died of tuberculosis. At autopsy, he found four small tumors in the submucosa of the ileum, with similar features to those previously described: nests of cells with dense, fibrous connective disuse. The second case was a young woman who died of typhoid fever; there were three small tumors in the ileum, all spaced far away from each other. He had four more cases displaying similar findings; he observed that there were multiple primary malignant tumors in the same organ. Oberndorfer concluded that these tumors were not true carcinoma; they grew slowly, had sharp borders, and did not metastasize. He felt these odd tumors could not be grouped with carcinoma of the small bowel, so he termed the "carcinoma-like," hence the term carcinoid. Unfortunately, Oberndorfer's initial descriptions of carcinoid did not encompass the true nature of the disease. It would be 22 years later that he would describe 36 more carcinoids of the appendix and small intestine.[49] In those cases, he revised his initial assessment to include the fact that the tumors were malignant and had the potential to metastasize.

Further characterization of these tumors would rely on the new techniques being developed in microscopy. First described in 1868, enterochromaffin cells of the gastric mucosa were nothing more than a microscopic observation.[50] In 1897, Nikolai Kulchitsky found similar staining cells in the crypts of Lieberkuhn.[11,51,52] However, it was not until 1914 that Pierre Masson applied silver stains to carcinoid tumors.[53] In his first description of an appendiceal carcinoid, he used saffron and trichrome stains to observe a polarization of their secretory vesicles.[54] From that, he deduced that the carcinoid tumor was actually an endocrine neoplasm and that chromaffin cells were the origin.[55] Fourteen years later, Masson described enterochromaffin cells to be of neural origin and stated that they could secrete substances. While the actual description of the carcinoid syndrome would not be documented until a few years later, the microscopic cellular findings correlated well with clinic findings.

The collection of symptoms known as the carcinoid syndrome commonly includes flushing, diarrhea, and edema. It was first formally described by Scholte, who documented an ileal carcinoid in a 47-year-old man who suffered from diarrhea, cyanosis, cough, and lower extremity edema, who eventually died of heart failure and bronchopneumonia.[56] At autopsy, it was also noted that he had hard thickening of the tricuspid valve and irregular endocardial thickening of the right atrium. This report was the first documentation of carcinoid heart disease. Over the next 20 years, more cases were published describing the syndrome with associated metastatic carcinoid. It was also during this period, in 1948, that Rappoport first isolated and described serotonin.[57] In 1954, Thorson and colleagues published the first series of patients presenting with pulmonary stenosis, tricuspid insufficiency, peripheral vasomotor symptoms, bronchoconstriction, and cyanosis in association with malignant carcinoid tumor of the small intestine with metastases to the liver.[58] In the initial report, they presented seven definite cases, four probable cases, and five with partial or not fully verified symptoms. In the same year, Pernow and Waldenström added paroxysmal flushing as a key component of this syndrome.[59] Soon after, serotonin was isolated from enterochromaffin cells and eventually from an ileal carcinoid, proving that enterochromaffin cells actually contained this bioactive amine. Lembeck confirmed in 1953 biochemically the presence of serotonin in an ileal carcinoid tumor, thus concluding that human EC-cells contained this bioactive ammine.[60] In 1966, Anthony Pearse recognized that the endocrine cells of the gut were linked together by a group of common cytochemical characteristics, in particular, the uptake of 5-hydroxytryptophan and its decarboxylation to 5-HT.[61] By 1968, these peptide hormone-producing cells, all of which derived from the neural crest, were collectively entitled APUD (amine precursor uptake and decarboxylation) cells, although more recently this acronym has been modified somewhat and is referred to as the diffuse neuroendocrine system (DNES).[62] While Pearse and others initially suggested that APUD cells were derived from neural crest cells, it is now generally recognized that GEP APUD cells probably arise from endoderm. Le Dourain and colleagues subsequently demonstrated that multipotency of neural crest cells and proposed that enteric gangliogenesis by neural crest cells reflected the effects of multiple growth factors of the glial-derived neurotrophic factor family.[63,64]

THE BIRTH OF THE DIFFUSE ENDOCRINE SYSTEM, ITS HORMONES, AND ITS DISEASES

This evolving concept of a diffuse endocrine system continued to mature and was first formally described by Feyrter in 1938.[65] By summing up decades of work on secretory organs and cells, he recognized that the endocrine system consisted of traditional compact epithelial organs as well as scattered cells either individually or in groups. These cells could be seen not only in the pancreas, but also throughout the gut. He additionally recognized that these cells were connected within the neural network of the gut wall. This structural relationship existed within the adrenal cortex and medulla, supporting a general and anatomically integrated model of the neuroendocrine system.

Famous syndromes would arise from the cells of the neuroendocrine system. The adrenal glands were described in the 16th century, but it was not for another 300 years that their importance was appreciated. In 1855, Addison described 12 patients with adrenal disorders, some who died of adrenal deficiency (Addison disease).[7] In 1912, Cushing described a patient with weight gain, muscle weakness, back pain, irregular menstruations, a round face, hypertrichosis, hyperpigmentation, and extensive bleeding with hypertension (Cushing syndrome).[66] Eventually, this patient was recognized to have hypercortism, and she was treated with a craniotomy and removal of the pituitary.

In 1927, Wilder described a case of insulin-secreting tumor, and later Whipple described the clinical picture of hyperinsulinism.[67,68] In 1948, glucagon was isolated by Sutherland and de Duve, although some years previously Becker described probably the first glucagon-secreting tumor.[69,70] The glucagonoma syndrome was well documented by McGavran in 1966.[71] In 1946, an ulcerogenic syndrome associated with a pancreatic islet cell tumor was described for the first time, and in 1955, Zollinger and Ellison provided details of the syndrome that still carries their names.[72] It was not until 1964, however, that Gregory and Tracy isolated gastrin.[73] In 1958, a description was given of a diarrheogenic syndrome related to an endocrine tumor of the pancreas by Verner and Morrison.[74] This was many years before the hormone responsible vasoactive intestinal polypeptide (VIP) was isolated.[75] The identification of different inherited multiple endocrine adenomatoses syndrome was due to Wermer, Sipple and Williams, and Pollock in 1954, 1961, and 1966 respectively.[76–78]

Until 1960, most of the well-known clinical syndromes related to release of substances from the gastro-pancreatic tract were described, although the exact mediators were not delineated. Following the initial slow development in the recognition of GEP peptides/amines, there was an exponential rate of growth of discoveries in relation to advances in protein chemistry that led to isolation and characterization of more than 50 GEP peptides. An increased awareness of the actions of these hormones, coupled with improved methods of detection, led to the recognition of the role of these peptides in physiology and pathophysiology, and many tumor-associated syndromes were predicted to overproduction of one or more GEP peptides/amines. The late 1960s to early 1970s was the era of detection of a lot of new GEP peptides/amines, particularly by work from Mutt and Jorpes from Stockholm. Viktor Mutt was boiling tons of pig intestines and thereby could extract peptides, such as VIP, GIP, PYY, and so forth.[79] This was the golden era of GEP peptides.

SCIENCE CHANGES: INSULIN AND THE RIA

The disease known today as diabetes mellitus was well described in ancient times. The symptoms of polyuria, polydipsia, and subsequent death were known to be associated with sweet urine by ancient Egyptians, Indians, and Greeks. In fact, the term for diabetes in the Chinese language is literally, sweet urine disease. The measurement of documentation of diabetes has evolved over the centuries. Consistently, physicians made the diagnosis by tasting the urine. It became somewhat more objective when the ancient Chinese and Indians tested a patient's urine to see if it was sweet enough to attract ants. Banting and Best, in their famous dog experiments, were able to measure blood glucose levels and urine glucose to nitrogen ratios to document diabetes. However, a revolutionary technique was developed that would change the way scientists could measure extremely small quantities of biologically interesting molecules, all from insulin.

Insulin measurements are a relatively trivial technique by today's standards, but in the early 20th century, normal insulin levels in the blood were not defined. The only tools available at the time were biologic; an extract of tissue or serum was injected into a depancreatized, adrenalectomized, or hypophysectomized animal, and the drop in blood glucose was used as the outcome.[80] This method had poor accuracy, precision, reproducibility, and sensitivity. Moreover, it usually required large amounts of serum to get any type of effect. Other assays were developed involving rat diaphragm muscle or epididymal fat pads and their glucose uptake.[81,82] However, in addition to the previously mentioned problems, these tests were also influenced by insulin-like molecules that could change blood glucose metabolism. These problems were solved by the RIA.[83]

Rosalyn Yalow and Solomon Berson settled in the New York area and worked together at the Brown Veterans Administration Hospital in the Radioisotope Unit: Yalow the scientist, Berson the physician. They started their studies with ^{131}I-labelled insulin and its metabolism in diabetes. They were able to show that people with diabetes treated with insulin always produced anti-insulin antibodies. These antibodies would be well characterized, but they would also be used as a tool. Yalow and Berson recognized that this competitive binding of an unknown amount of unlabelled insulin with a known amount of radiolabeled insulin to a known amount of antibody could accurately measure the amount of insulin, even in a vast mixture of other molecules. The discovery of RIA was published in 1960 and led to a Nobel Prize in 1977.[43] More importantly, it provided the basis of measuring small quantities of other hormones. It supported earlier theories that there were two major types of diabetes, one insulin-deficient (type 1 diabetes) and one insulin-resistant (type 2 diabetes). Studies based on RIA also showed that insulin resistance was associated with obesity, gestational diabetes, acromegaly, and Cushing disease.[84,85] While confusing at first, other insulin-like molecules eventually would be described (IGF-1 and IGF-2). RIA also was used as an important tool to study membrane receptors, which previously were difficult to detect and quantify. Eventually, this technique would be the standard to measure proteins, peptides, and other molecules in all fields of medicine.

FROM BRAIN TO GUT: SOMATOSTATIN

The history of somatostatin left an indelible mark on the central and digestive nervous systems. While its discovery was not as dramatic as insulin, the story of somatostatin is tightly woven with insulin, and their paths cross throughout endocrine history. In its own right, somatostatin has many powerful physiologic effects and is used by many cell types with diverse biologic effects.

The story of somatostatin begins in the brain, where growth hormone (GH) was an important topic of research. It was well known that GH was expressed by pituitary and had profound peripheral effects. What was unknown in the 1960s was how GH was regulated. In 1964, GH-releasing hormone (GHRH) was isolated from the stalk–median eminences of sheep hypothalamus.[86] During the column purification of GHRH, another fraction contained a substance that had inhibitory effects on growth hormone release—a GH-inhibiting factor (GIF). In 1968, Krulich and colleagues isolated from rat hypothalamus a substance with an inhibiting action of the release of pituitary GH and called it GH RIF.[87] In the same year, Hellman and Lernmark reported on the presence of a potent inhibitor of insulin secretion in extracts of pancreatic islets.[88] Eventually, GIF would be isolated and purified from 500,000 sheep hypothalami by Guillemin and Brasseau using a new in vitro assay in 1973.[89,90] As multiple groups competed for its discovery and characterization, it went through many names, including GIF, somatotropin release-inhibiting factor (SRIF), panhibin, and somatostatin. Shortly after its discovery and characterization, the structure of somatostatin was solved and allowed it to be purified and synthesized.[91] Using RIA and immunohistochemistry methods, it was shown that somatostatin-like immunoreactivity was heterogeneously distributed in tissue of many animal species, vertebrate as well as in vertebrates. The first somatostatin-producing neoplasm of the endocrine pancreas was described in 1977 by Larsson and colleagues, and the clinical presentation included diabetes mellitus, gallbladder disease, anemia, delayed gastric emptying, and loss of weight.[92] Somatostatin inhibits the secretion of several gut hormones (eg, insulin and glucagon) and digestive events, such as stomach acid and pancreatic fluid secretion. The discovery of somatostatin and its effects would be rewarded with a Nobel Prize in 1977 to Roger Guillemin and Andrew Schally, the same year as Rosalyn Yalow.

It was in mid 1970s that the history of somatostatin mixed with that of insulin.[38] Up until this time, insulin was purified from porcine pancreas, but injections were painful and often associated with bad reactions. The race to produce a synthetic insulin absorbed the time of multiple groups in the United States. Some groups chose to produce it as a recombinant protein in genetically altered bacteria, but another group chose a chemical route. Keiichi Itakura, Herbert Boyer, and Arthur Riggs set forth to chemically construct a whole gene and implant it into a bacteria to produce a recombinant human insulin. However, before they could tackle a gene the size of insulin, they chose to test their technique on a much smaller protein, somatostatin. Itakura chemically synthesized a gene that would code for the 14 amino acid long peptide and implant

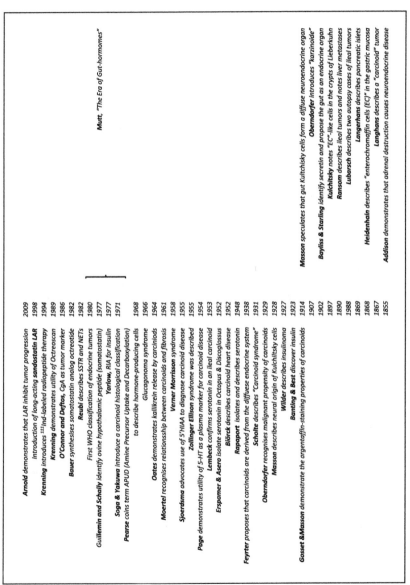

Fig. 1. The historical development of the gastroenteropancreatic endocrine axis.

it into *Eshcerichia coli*.[93] The experiment worked. Unlike their competitors, who were facing major public and political resistance to putting human genes into bacteria, Itakura, Boyer, and Riggs saw no conflict in their chemical gene. This technology gave birth to the pharmaceutical company Genentech. It was a short step to scaling up the procedure to produce insulin. Thus, somatostatin was the first recombinant human peptide ever synthesized in large quantities by bacterial recombination.

In 1978, Vale and Riviere reported on an octapeptide analog that displayed the full biologic activity of somatostatin, and from 1980 to 1982, Bauer and colleagues at Sandoz synthesized an analog named octreotide.[94,95] Shortly thereafter, other companies and research institutes became interested in somatostatin analogs and produced several other analogs, such as lanreotide and RC160, and most recently SOM230 (Pasireotide by Novartis). Five somatostatin receptor subtypes (SSTR1-SSTR5) have been identified by gene cloning techniques.[96] These subtypes also differ in their binding affinity to specific somatostatin analogs, an important characteristic relevant to imaging and therapeutics. All somatostatin receptor subtypes are G-protein coupled receptors.

In 1982, Reubi and colleagues reported on the expression of somatostatin receptor type 2 in neuroendocrine tumors (NETs).[97,98] In 1983, the first somatostatin analogs were used in clinical practice for treatment of severe clinical symptoms related to NETs, such as carcinoid syndrome, the Verner Morrison syndrome, and glucagonoma syndrome.[99] Since then, the synthetic analog of somatostatin, octreotide (Sandostatin), proved to be an excellent therapy to control the symptoms from NETs, and convenient to administer (one injection every 4 weeks). Somatostatin receptor was also a powerful target in NET diagnostics. In 1989, somatostatin receptor scintigraphy was introduced by Krenning and his research group in Holland and later in the beginning of 1990s, Krenning's group introduced tumor targeted radioactive treatment (PRRT) with radiolabeled somatostatin analogs for treatment.[100,101] In the beginning[111] indium-labeled, later on ^{90}yttrium, and finally ^{177}lutetium-DOTA-octreotate were applied in the treatment of various NETs.[102–105] Today therapy with somatostatin analogs is the gold standard for patients with functioning tumors. Somatostatin scintigraphy is a working horse in the management of neuroendocrine tumors. It will soon be replaced by positron emission tomography using ^{68}gallium-DOTA-octreotate.[106]

From 1980 to 1990, new peptides were identified, which could be used as tumor markers in GEP-NETs. The authors' group reported on the expression of tachykinins in carcinoid tumors in 1984.[107] In 1986, O'Connor and Deftos described the use of chromogranin A as a general tumor marker in peptide-producing endocrine neoplasms.[108] This marker is now the gold standard for diagnosis and follow-up of different types of neuroendocrine tumors. Chromogranin A is a member of the chromogranin family, stored in secretory granules of 80% of all NETs. The latest described clinical syndrome related to GEP-NET was published from the authors' group in 2004.[109] It was a patient with a ghrelin-producing tumor of the gut. Ghrelin-producing tumors have been published from other groups involving the pancreas and stomach. Many NETs can ectopically produce other hormones such as ACTH, GRP, calcitonin, HCG-α and PTH-RP. A summary is found in **Fig. 1**.

SUMMARY

For those with an interest in the GEP axis, its history is as compelling and fascinating as the hormones themselves. When a patient complains of flushing and diarrhea, those were the same complaints seen by Oberdorffer. When a young person with newly diagnosed diabetes starts insulin, it is the same miracle treatment discovered by Banting and Best. When a NET is treated with somatostatin analog, it is thanks to chemists and biologists that it can be injected just once a month. Over the decades, GEP hormone research has been recognized at the highest levels, not only for its effects on patients, but its effects on science. As long as there are still patients who struggle with GEP diseases, there will still be more history to write.

REFERENCES

1. Modlin IM, Champaneria MC, Bornschein J, et al. Evolution of the diffuse neuro-endocrine system—clear cells and cloudy origins. Neuroendocrinology 2006; 84(2):69–82.
2. Himes NE. Medical history of contraception. Medical aspects of human fertility series issued by the National Committee on Maternal Health, Inc. Baltimore (MD): The Williams & Wilkins Company; 1936. p. 521.
3. Harris GW. Humours and hormones. J Endocrinol 1972;53(2):2–23.
4. Sharpey-Schafer E. Endocrine physiology. Ir J Med Sci 1931;69:483–505.
5. Bernard C. Sur une nouvelle fonction du foie chez l'homme et les animaux [A new function of the liver of humans and animals]. CR Acad Sci 1850;31: 571–4 [in French].
6. Hunter J. Observations on certain parts of the animal oeconomy 1786. London.
7. Addison T. On the constitution and local effects of diseases of the supra renal capsules. London: Samuel Highley; 1855.
8. Kocher T. Concerning pathological manifestations in low-grade thyroid diseases. In Proceedings from Nobel Lectures 1909.
9. Brown-Sequard C. Recherches experimentales sur la physiologie et la patholo-gie des capsules surrenales. CR Acad Sci 1856;43:422–5 [in French].
10. Langerhans P. Beitrage zur mikdroskopischen Anatomie der Bauchspeichel-druse [Microscopical anatomy of the pancreas]. Berlin; 1869 [in German]
11. Kulchitsky N. Zur Frage uber den Bau des Darmkanals [Question about the construction of the intestinal tract]. Arch Mikr Anat 1897;49:7–35 [in German].
12. Pavlov I. Die Innervation des Pankreas [The innervation of pancreas]. Klin Wochenzeitung 1888;32:667–75 [in German].
13. Pavlov I. Lektsii o rabote glavnykh pischchevaritel'nykh zhelez [The innervation of pancreas]. St Petersburg, Russia: Piroda; 1897.
14. Pavlov IP. Lectures on the work of the digestive glands. London: Charles Griffin and Company; 1910.
15. Modlin IM. From Prout to the proton pump—a history of the science of gastric acid secretion and the surgery of peptic ulcer. Surg Gynecol Obstet 1990; 170(1):81–96.
16. Modlin IM, Kidd M. Ernest Starling and the discovery of secretin. J Clin Gastro-enterol 2001;32(3):187–92.
17. Martin C. Ernest Henry Starling: life and work. BMJ 1927;1:900–4.
18. Bayliss WM, Starling EH. The mechanism of pancreatic secretion. J Physiol 1902;28:325–52.
19. Hirst BH. Secretin and the exposition of hormonal control. J Physiol 2004;560(2): 339.
20. Starling E. The Croonian lectures on the chemical correlation of the functions of the body. Lancet 1905;166:339–41.
21. Edkins J. The chemical mechanism of gastric secretion. J Physiol 1906;34:133–44.
22. Langley JA, Anderson HK. On reflex action from sympathetic ganglia. J Physiol 1894;16:410–40.
23. Elliot T. On the action of adrenaline. J Physiol 1904;31:10–21.

24. Bliss M. The discovery of insulin. Chicago: University of Chicago Press; 1982.
25. LeRoith D, Taylor SI, Olefsky JM. Diabetes mellitus: a fundamental and clinical text. 3rd edition. Philadelphia: Lippincott Williams & Wilkins; 2004.
26. Gemmill CL. The Greek concept of diabetes. Bull N Y Acad Med 1972;48(8): 1033–6.
27. Papaspyros NS. The history of diabetes mellitus. London: Robert Stockwell Limited; 1952.
28. Frank LL. Diabetes mellitus in the texts of old Hindu medicine (Charaka, Susruta, Vagbhata). Am J Gastroenterol 1957;27(1):76–95.
29. Ahmed AM. History of diabetes mellitus. Saudi Med J 2002;23(4):373–8.
30. Eisenbarth GS, Connelly J, Soeldner JS. The natural history of type 1 diabetes. Diabetes Metab Rev 1987;3(4):873–91.
31. Allen FM. Experimental studies on diabetes: series I. Production and control of diabetes in the dog. 4. Control of experimental diabetes by fasting and total dietary restriction. J Exp Med 1920;31(5):575–86.
32. Blades M, Morgan JB, Dickerson JW. Dietary advice in the management of diabetes mellitus—history and current practice. J R Soc Health 1997;117(3):143–50.
33. Cox C. The fight to survive: a young girl, diabetes, and the discovery of insulin. New York: Kaplan Publishing; 2009.
34. Joslin EP. The treatment of diabetes mellitus: with observations upon the disease based upon thirteen hundred cases. 2nd edition. Philadelphia: Lea & Febiger; 1917.
35. Bliss M. Banting: a biography. Toronto: McClelland and Stewart; 1984.
36. Banting FB, Best CH, MacLeod JJR. The internal secretion of the pancreas. Am J Physiol 1922;59:479.
37. Banting FB, Best CH, Collip JB, et al. The effect of pancreatic extract (insulin) on normal rabbits. Am J Physiol 1922;62:559–80.
38. Hall SS. Invisible frontiers: the race to synthesize a human gene. New York: Oxford University Press; 2002.
39. Sanger F, Tuppy H. The amino acid sequence in the phenylalanyl chain of insulin. I. The identification of lower peptides from partial hydrolysates. Biochem J 1951; 49(4):463–81.
40. Hodgkin DC. The Banting memorial lecture 1972. The structure of insulin. Diabetes 1972;21(12):1131–50.
41. Harding MM, Hodgkin DC, Kennedy AF, et al. The crystal structure of insulin. II. An investigation of rhombohedral zinc insulin crystals and a report of other crystalline forms. J Mol Biol 1966;16(1):212–26.
42. Dodson E, Harding MM, Hodgkin DC, et al. The crystal structure of insulin. 3. Evidence for a 2-fold axis in rhombohedral zinc insulin. J Mol Biol 1966;16(1):227–41.
43. Yalow RS, Berson SA. Immunoassay of endogenous plasma insulin in man. J Clin Invest 1960;39:1157–75.
44. Modlin IM, Shapiro MD, Kidd M. Siegfried Oberndorfer: origins and perspectives of carcinoid tumors. Hum Pathol 2004;35(12):1440–51.
45. Langhans T. Über einen Drusenpolyp im Ileum [Report on a glandular polyp in ileum]. Virchows Arch Pathol Anat Physiol Klin Med 1867;38:550–60 [in German].
46. Lubarsch O. Über dem primaren Krebs des Ileum nebst bemerkungen über das gleichzeitige Vorkommen von Krebs und Tuberculose [About the primary cancer of the ileum, together with remarks about the simultaneous occurrence of cancer and tuberculosis]. Virchows Arch 1888;111:280–317 [in German].
47. Ransom W. A case of primary carcinoma of the ileum. Lancet 1890;2:1020–3.

48. Oberndorfer S. Karzinoid Tumoren des Dunndarms [Carcinoid tumors in the small intestine]. Frankf Z Pathol 1907;1:426–32 [in French].
49. Oberndorfer S. Karzinoide Handbuch der Speziellen [Special carcinoid handbook]. In: Henke FL, Lubarsch O, editors. Handbuch der Speziellen Pathologischen Anatomie und Histologie. Berlin: Verlag von Julius Springer; 1928. p. 814–47 [in German].
50. Heidenhain R. Untersuchungen uber den Bau der Labdrusen [Investigation of the construction of the 'Lab gland']. Arch Mikr Anat 1870;6:368 [in German].
51. Drozdov I, Modlin IM, Kidd M, et al. From Leningrad to London: the saga of Kulchitsky and the legacy of the enterochromaffin cell. Neuroendocrinology 2009;89(1):1–12.
52. Drozdov I, Modlin IM, Kidd M, et al. Nikolai Konstantinovich Kulchitsky (1856–1925). J Med Biogr 2009;17(1):47–54.
53. Gosset AM, Masson P. Tumeurs endocrines de l'appendice [Endocrine tumors of the appendix]. Presse Med 1914;25:237–40 [in French].
54. Steffen C. The man behind the eponym: C.L. Pierre Masson. Am J Dermatopathol 2003;25(1):71–6.
55. Michalany I. Masson's contribution to pathology and to histological technique. With special reference to the discovery of argentaffin cells. Ann Pathol 1983; 3(1):85–93.
56. Scholte A. Ein Fall von Angioma teleangiectaticum cutis mit chronischer Endocarditis und Malignem dunndarmcarcinoid [One case of skin teleangiectasies and chronic endocarditis and malignant small intestinal carcionoid]. Beitr Pathol Anat 1931;86:440–3 [in German].
57. Rapport MM, Green AA, Page IH. Partial purification of the vasoconstrictor in beef serum. J Biol Chem 1948;174(2):735–41.
58. Thorson A, Biorck G, Bjorkman G, et al. Malignant carcinoid of the small intestine with metastases to the liver, valvular disease of the right side of the heart (pulmonary stenosis and tricuspid regurgitation without septal defects), peripheral vasomotor symptoms, bronchoconstriction, and an unusual type of cyanosis; a clinical and pathologic syndrome. Am Heart J 1954;47(5):795–817.
59. Pernow B, Waldenstrom J. Paroxysmal flushing and other symptoms caused by 5-hydroxytryptamine and histamine in patients with malignant tumours. Lancet 1954;267(6845):951.
60. Lembeck F. 5-Hydroxytryptamine in a carcinoid tumour. Nature 1953;172:910–1.
61. Pearse AG. 5-Hydroxytryptophan uptake by dog thyroid 'C' cells, and its possible significance in polypeptide hormone production. Nature 1966; 211(5049):598–600.
62. Pearse AG. The diffuse endocrine system and the implications of the APUD concept. Int Surg 1979;64(2):5–7.
63. Le Douarin NM. On the origin of pancreatic endocrine cells. Cell 1988;53(2): 169–71.
64. Le Douarin NM, Dupin E. Multipotentiality of the neural crest. Curr Opin Genet Dev 2003;13(5):529–36.
65. Feyrter F. Über diffuse Endokrine epitheliale Organe [Presentation of the diffuse endocrine system]. Zentralbl Innere Med 1938;545:31–41 [in German].
66. Cushing H. The pituitary body and its disorders. Philadelphia: Lippincott Company; 1912.
67. Wilder RA, Allan FN, Power MF, et al. Carcinoma of the islands of the pancreas. Hyperinsulinism and hypoglycemia. J Am Med Assoc 1927;89:48.
68. Whipple AF, Frantz VK. Adenoma of islet cells with hyperinsulinism, a review. Ann Surg 1935;101:1299.

69. Sutherland EW, De Duve C. Origin and distribution of the hyperglycemic–glycogenolytic factor of the pancreas. J Biol Chem 1948;175:663–74.

70. Becker SK, Kahn D, Rothman S. Cutaneous manifestations of internal malignant tumors. Arch Derm Syphilol 1942;45:1069–80.

71. McGavran MH, Unger RH, Recant L, et al. A glucagon-secreting alpha-cell carcinoma of the pancreas. N Engl J Med 1966;274(25):1408–13.

72. Zollinger RM, Ellison EH. Primary peptic ulcerations of the jejunum associated with islet cell tumors of the pancreas. Ann Surg 1955;142(4):709–23 [discussion: 724–8].

73. Tracy HJ, Gregory RA. Physiological properties of a series of synthetic peptides structurally related to gastrin I. Nature 1964;204:935–8.

74. Verner JV, Morrison AB. Islet cell tumor and a syndrome of refractory watery diarrhea and hypokalemia. Am J Med 1958;25(3):374–80.

75. Said SI, Mutt V. Isolation from porcine-intestinal wall of a vasoactive octacosapeptide related to secretin and to glucagon. Eur J Biochem 1972;28(2):199–204.

76. Wermer P. Genetic aspects of adenomatosis of endocrine glands. Am J Med 1954;16(3):363–71.

77. Sipple J. The association of pheochromocytoma with carinoma of the thyroid gland. Am J Med 1961;31:163–6.

78. Williams ED, Pollock DJ. Multiple mucosal neuromata with endocrine tumours: a syndrome allied to von Recklinghausen's disease. J Pathol Bacteriol 1966; 91(1):71–80.

79. Gozes I. In memory of Victor Mutt. Discoveries of biologically important peptides. J Mol Neurosci 1998;11(2):105–8.

80. Gellhorn EF, Allen A. Assay of insulin on hypophysectomized, adreno-demedullated, and hypophysectomized-adreno-demedulated rats. Endocrinology 1941; 29:137–40.

81. Groen J, Kamminga CE, Willebrands AF, et al. Evidence for the presence of insulin in blood serum; a method for an approximate determination of the insulin content of blood. J Clin Invest 1952;31(1):97–106.

82. Renold AE, Martin DB, Dagenais YM, et al. Measurement of small quantities of insulin-like activity using rat adipose tissue. I. A proposed procedure. J Clin Invest 1960;39:1487–98.

83. Kahn CR, Roth J. Berson, Yalow, and the JCI: the agony and the ecstasy. J Clin Invest 2004;114(8):1051–4.

84. Yalow RS. Radioimmunoassay: a probe for the fine structure of biologic systems. Science 1978;200(4347):1236–45.

85. Yalow RS, Glick SM, Roth J, et al. Plasma insulin and growth hormone levels in obesity and diabetes. Ann N Y Acad Sci 1965;131(1):357–73.

86. Deuben RR, Meites J. Stimulation of pituitary growth hormone release by a hypothalamic extract in vitro. Endocrinology 1964;74:408–14.

87. Krulich L, Dhariwal AP, McCann SM. Stimulatory and inhibitory effects of purified hypothalamic extracts on growth hormone release from rat pituitary in vitro. Endocrinology 1968;83(4):783–90.

88. Hellman B, Lernmark A. Evidence for an inhibitor of insulin release in the pancreatic islets. Diabetologia 1969;5(1):22–4.

89. Vale W, Grant G, Rivier J, et al. Synthetic polypeptide antagonists of the hypothalamic luteinizing hormone releasing factor. Science 1972;176(37):933–4.

90. Brazeau P, Vale W, Burgus R, et al. Hypothalamic polypeptide that inhibits the secretion of immunoreactive pituitary growth hormone. Science 1973;179(68): 77–9.

91. Burgus R, Ling N, Butcher M, et al. Primary structure of somatostatin, a hypothalamic peptide that inhibits the secretion of pituitary growth hormone. Proc Natl Acad Sci U S A 1973;70(3):684–8.
92. Larsson LI, Hirsch MA, Holst JJ, et al. Pancreatic somatostatinoma. Clinical features and physiological implications. Lancet 1977;1(8013):666–8.
93. Itakura K, Hirose T, Crea R, et al. Expression in *Escherichia coli* of a chemically synthesized gene for the hormone somatostatin. Science 1977;198(4321): 1056–63.
94. Vale W, Rivier J, Ling N, et al. Biologic and immunologic activities and applications of somatostatin analogs. Metabolism 1978;27:1391–401.
95. Pless J. From somatostatin to sandostatin: history and chemistry. Digestion 1993;54(Suppl 1):7–8.
96. Tulipano G, Schulz S. Novel insights in somatostatin receptor physiology. Eur J Endocrinol 2007;156(Suppl 1):S3–11.
97. Reubi JC, Rivier J, Perrin M, et al. Specific high-affinity binding sites for somatostatin-28 on pancreatic beta-cells: differences with brain somatostatin receptors. Endocrinology 1982;110(3):1049–51.
98. Reubi JC, Maurer R, von Werder K, et al. Somatostatin receptors in human endocrine tumors. Cancer Res 1987;47(2):551–8.
99. Bauer W, Briner U, Doepfner W, et al. SMS 201–995: a very potent and selective octapeptide analogue of somatostatin with prolonged action. Life Sci 1982; 31(11):1133–40.
100. Lamberts SW, Bakker WH, Reubi JC, et al. Somatostatin-receptor imaging in the localization of endocrine tumors. N Engl J Med 1990;323(18):1246–9.
101. Krenning EP, Kooij PP, Bakker WH, et al. Radiotherapy with a radiolabeled somatostatin analogue, [111In-DTPA-D-Phe1]-octreotide. A case history. Ann N Y Acad Sci 1994;733:496–506.
102. Fjalling M, Andersson P, Forssell-Aronsson E, et al. Systemic radionuclide therapy using indium-111-DTPA-D-Phe1-octreotide in midgut carcinoid syndrome. J Nucl Med 1996;37(9):1519–21.
103. Bushnell DL Jr, O'Dorisio TM, O'Dorisio MS, et al. 90Y-edotreotide for metastatic carcinoid refractory to octreotide. J Clin Oncol 2010;28(10):1652–9.
104. Waldherr C, Pless M, Maecke HR, et al. Tumor response and clinical benefit in neuroendocrine tumors after 7.4 GBq (90)Y-DOTATOC. J Nucl Med 2002;43(5): 610–6.
105. Kwekkeboom DJ, de Herder WW, Kam BL, et al. Treatment with the radiolabeled somatostatin analog [177 Lu-DOTA 0, Tyr3]octreotate: toxicity, efficacy, and survival. J Clin Oncol 2008;26(13):2124–30.
106. Kowalski J, Henze M, Schuhmacher J, et al. Evaluation of positron emission tomography imaging using [68Ga]-DOTA-D Phe(1)-Tyr(3)-Octreotide in comparison to [111In]-DTPAOC SPECT. First results in patients with neuroendocrine tumors. Mol Imaging Biol 2003;5(1):42–8.
107. Norheim I, Theodorsson-Norheim E, Brodin E, et al. Antisera raised against eledoisin and kassinin detect elevated levels of immunoreactive material in plasma and tumor tissues from patients with carcinoid tumors. Regul Pept 1984;9(4):245–57.
108. O'Connor DT, Deftos LJ. Secretion of chromogranin A by peptide-producing endocrine neoplasms. N Engl J Med 1986;314(18):1145–51.
109. Tsolakis AV, Portela-Gomes GM, Stridsberg M, et al. Malignant gastric ghrelinoma with hyperghrelinemia. J Clin Endocrinol Metab 2004;89(8):3739–44.

Pathology of Gastrointestinal Disorders

Guido Rindi, MD, PhD[a],*, Frediano Inzani, MD[a,b], Enrico Solcia, MD[b]

KEYWORDS

- Hyperplasia • Dysplasia • Neoplasia • Carcinoid
- Neuroendocrine tumor • Neuroendocrine carcinoma

This review aims to provide a brief description of nonneoplastic and neoplastic endocrine growths of the gastrointestinal tract according to an anatomic approach (**Tables 1–3**). Each section details specific diagnostic and relevant clinical aspects.

STOMACH
Hyperplasia-dysplasia

Gastric endocrine cell proliferation is observed in conditions of long-standing hypergastrinemia (see **Table 1**). The most common underlying conditions are: (1) achlorhydria associated with chronic atrophic gastritis (CAG); (2) functioning gastrin producing tumors (gastrinoma) in Zollinger-Ellison syndrome (ZES), either with or without the multiple endocrine neoplasia syndrome type 1 (MEN1); and (3) long-term proton-pump inhibitor (PPI) treatment.[1–4] Enterochromaffin-like (ECL) cell tumors (carcinoids) develop in 13% to 43% of patients with MEN1 compared with less than 1% in patients with ZES without MEN1.[1]

Corpus-fundus

Proliferative lesions of endocrine cells of the stomach are categorized, in terms of severity and capacity to progress to well-differentiated endocrine tumors (carcinoids), for ECL cells only.[5] Other endocrine cells, such as enterochromaffin (EC) and ghrelin cells, may also be involved as minor populations.[2,6–11] Hypergastrinemia drives ECL cell hyperplasia to dysplasia and neoplasia via a multistep process.[1,5,12–14]

The authors have nothing to disclose.

[a] Institute of Anatomic Pathology, Università Cattolica del Sacro Cuore – Policlinico A. Gemelli, Largo A. Gemelli, 8, Rome I-00168, Italy

[b] Department of Human Pathology and Heredity, University of Pavia, via Forlanini 16, 27100 Pavia, Italy

* Corresponding author.

E-mail address: guido.rindi@rm.unicatt.it

Endocrinol Metab Clin N Am 39 (2010) 713–727

doi:10.1016/j.ecl.2010.08.009

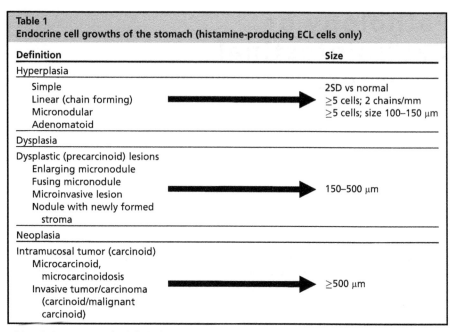

Table 1
Endocrine cell growths of the stomach (histamine-producing ECL cells only)

Definition	Size
Hyperplasia	
Simple	2SD vs normal
Linear (chain forming)	≥5 cells; 2 chains/mm
Micronodular	≥5 cells; size 100–150 μm
Adenomatoid	
Dysplasia	
Dysplastic (precarcinoid) lesions	
Enlarging micronodule	
Fusing micronodule	
Microinvasive lesion	150–500 μm
Nodule with newly formed stroma	
Neoplasia	
Intramucosal tumor (carcinoid)	
Microcarcinoid, microcarcinoidosis	
Invasive tumor/carcinoma (carcinoid/malignant carcinoid)	≥500 μm

Abbreviation: SD, standard deviation.
Data from Solcia E, Bordi C, Creutzfeldt W, et al. Histopathological classification of nonantral gastric endocrine growths in man. Digestion 1988;41:185–200.

ECL cell hyperplasia

Hyperplastic lesions lack tumor-progression potential and are classified as *simple* (*diffuse*), which has an increased number (more than 2 times greater than normal values) of endocrine cells; *linear or chain forming*, which has linear sequences of at least 5 cells along the basement membrane and at least 2 chains per millimeter length of mucosa; *micronodular*, which has clusters of 5 or more cells (30–150 μm) either within glands or in the lamina propria and at least 1 micronodule per millimeter length of mucosa; and *adenomatoid*, which is composed by at least 5 adjacent micronodules with intervening basal membrane within the lamina propria.

ECL cell dysplasia

These preneoplastic lesions sized between 150 to 500 μm display progressive similarity with tumors and are classified as *enlarging micronodules*, which have clusters of cells greater than 150 μm in size; *fusing micronodules*, which result from the disappearance of the basal membranes between adjacent micronodules; *microinvasive lesions*, which infiltrate the lamina propria and fill the space between glands; and *nodule with newly formed stroma,* which have a microlobular or trabecular structure.

Antrum

Antral gastrin (G) cell hyperplasia is the morphologic counterpart of hypergastrinemia, as usually observed in patients with hyperchlorhydria and gastric atrophy.[15,16] High numbers of G cells (140–250 per millimeter of mucosa vs 40–90 in controls) with palisades expanding toward the upper and lower portions of the antral glands usually associate with a reduction in somatostatin (D) cells and result in an abnormal G/D cell ratio.[17–22]

No dysplastic change of endocrine cells has been described in the antral mucosa.

Table 2
Gastrointestinal neoplasms with main cell types, their distribution in the gut, and possible associated hyperfunctional syndromes

| Tumor Type | Main Cell Type | Stomach | | | Intestine | | | | | | Syndrome |
| | | | | | Small | | | Large | | | |
		Pa	CF	An	D	J	I	Ap	C	R	
Well differentiated	B	+	⋮	⋮	⋮	⋮	⋮	⋮	⋮	⋮	Hypoglycemia
	A	+	⋮	⋮	⋮	⋮	⋮	⋮	⋮	⋮	Glucagonoma
	PP	+	⋮	⋮	⋮	⋮	⋮	⋮	⋮	⋮	-
	D	+	⋮	⋮	+	+	⋮	⋮	⋮	⋮	Somatostatinoma
	EC	+	+	+	+	+	+	+	+	+	Carcinoid
	ECL	⋮	+	⋮	⋮	⋮	⋮	⋮	⋮	⋮	Atypical carcinoid
	G	+	⋮	+	+	+	+	+	+	⋮	ZES
	L	⋮	⋮	⋮	+	+	+	+	+	+	-
	Ghrelin	+	+	⋮	⋮	⋮	⋮	⋮	⋮	⋮	(?)
Poorly differentiated[a]	S/L cells+	+	+	+	+	⋮	⋮	+	+	+	⋮

Abbreviations: An, antrum; Ap, appendix; C, colon; CF, corpus-fundus; D, duodenum; EC, enterochromaffin cell; ECL, enterochromaffin-like cell; I, ileum; J, jejunum; Pa, pancreas; R, rectum; S/L, small or large carcinoma cells; ZES, Zollinger-Ellison syndrome; +, presence of tumor; -, not defined.
[a] Poorly differentiated carcinomas are virtually never associated with hormonal syndromes.
Data from Rindi G, Villanacci V, Ubiali A, et al. Endocrine tumors of the digestive tract and pancreas: histogenesis, diagnosis and molecular basis. Expert Rev Mol Diagn 2001;1(3):323–33.

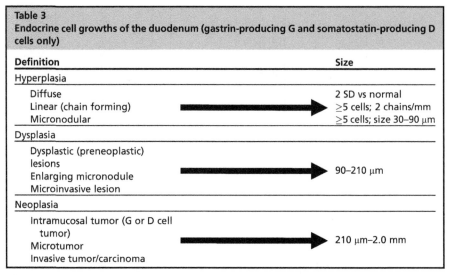

Table 3
Endocrine cell growths of the duodenum (gastrin-producing G and somatostatin-producing D cells only)

Definition	Size
Hyperplasia	
Diffuse	2 SD vs normal
Linear (chain forming)	≥5 cells; 2 chains/mm
Micronodular	≥5 cells; size 30–90 μm
Dysplasia	
Dysplastic (preneoplastic) lesions	
Enlarging micronodule	90–210 μm
Microinvasive lesion	
Neoplasia	
Intramucosal tumor (G or D cell tumor)	
Microtumor	210 μm–2.0 mm
Invasive tumor/carcinoma	

Abbreviation: SD, standard deviation.

Data from Anlauf M, Perren A, Meyer CL, et al. Precursor lesions in patients with multiple endocrine neoplasia type 1-associated duodenal gastrinomas. Gastroenterology 2005;128(5):1187–98; and Anlauf M, Perren A, Henopp T, et al. Allelic deletion of the MEN1 gene in duodenal gastrin and somatostatin cell neoplasms and their precursor lesions. Gut 2007;56(5):637–44.

Neoplasia

Tumor type

Well-differentiated neuroendocrine tumors (NETs) represent the largest fraction of gastric neuroendocrine neoplasms, with only a minority of high-grade, highly aggressive neuroendocrine carcinomas (NECs). Most NETs are made by tumor cells with ECL cell features.[23,24] Of 205 gastric neuroendocrine neoplasms, 193 (94%) were NETs with only 12 high-grade NECs, and 191 out of the 193 NETs (98%) were ECL cells NETs with only 2 G-cell NETs.[25] Rare EC cell tumors[26] and, more recently, 1 ghrelinoma have also been described (**Table 2**).[27]

Histology and grading

A 3-tiers grading system based on histology and proliferation was used to classify 102 gastric NETs.[28] Most cases (81/102) in this series, as well as in common practice, proved a monomorphic structure with solid nests and tubules, mild cellular atypia, and almost absent or few (0–2/10 high-power field [HPF]) typical mitoses. Prevalent solid aggregates, scant punctate necrosis, elevated mitotic count (≥7/10 HPF), and moderate cell atypia were observed in rare (5/102) gastric NETs. A total of 16 NECs showed solid structure, sometimes organoid, with diffuse geographic chart necrosis, small to intermediate, overtly atypical cells with numerous, often atypical, mitoses (**Fig. 1**B).[29] High-grade gastric NECs with medium size or even large cells have also been described.[30] The high-grade features and the frequent admixture with ordinary adenocarcinoma may lead to their misdiagnosis as poorly differentiated adenocarcinoma[31] or anaplastic carcinoma[32] with which they share the highest malignancy.[33] Based on the previous information, the grading system recently proposed by the European Neuroendocrine Tumor Society (ENETS) for gastrointestinal neuroendocrine neoplasms[28,34] proved effective in a series of 202 foregut neoplasms, 48 of which were gastric.[35] Its use is now supported by the American Joint Committee on Cancer.[36]

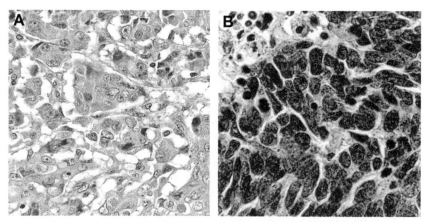

Fig. 1. Histology of gastrointestinal high-grade neuroendocrine carcinoma (NEC). (*A*) Organoid structure with sever atypical large cells in a NEC of the colon (large cell NEC): note the abundant eosinophilic cytoplasm with evident nucleoli; (*B*) Solid structure with necrosis (upper left corner) and small (fused) cell cytology in a NEC of the stomach (small cell NEC): note the salt and pepper chromatin, the scarce cytoplasm, inconspicuous nucleoli, and abundant mitoses; hematoxylin, and eosin.

Clinical settings

Three clinicopathologic types are described.[23,37] Type I ECL tumors associate with diffuse, corpus-restricted (A-type), A-CAG, achlorhydria, and hypergastrinemia; type II associate with hypergastrinemia and hypertrophic gastropathy caused by multiple endocrine neoplasia of type 1 and Zollinger-Ellison syndrome (MEN1-ZES); type III, or sporadic, do not associate with any distinctive gastric pathology or hypergastrinemia. A novel type IV was proposed for ECL cell NETs with achlorhydria, hypergastrinemia, corpus mucosa hypertrophy, and hyperplasia without MEN1-ZES.[38,39]

Type I ECL cell NETs, the most common, arise in the corpus fundus of aged patients, mainly women, are multiple and multicentric, small in size (usually <1 cm), and display well-differentiated G1 histology and associate with antral G-cell hyperplasia. Invasion of the muscularis propria is rare, metastases are exceptional, and survival usually excellent.[23,40] Type II ECL cell NETs are rare, display no sex prevalence,[25,41] and show histology features similar to type I. Local lymph node metastases have been reported, the survival is usually excellent. Nonetheless, an aggressive neoplasm with mixed G1 and G2/G3 histology was reported.[42,43] Type III ECL cell NETs, the second most common form, arise in younger men and are usually large and deeply invasive.[23,25,29] Histology may span from G1 to G2, including frequent mitoses, metastases (58% of 17),[29] and tumor-related death (7 of 26 subjects).[25]

High-grade NECs are aggressive, large (mean 4.2 cm, range 3.0–5.5) lesions, displaying deep-wall invasion, G3 histology, and a high proliferation rate ($\geq$20 mitotic count per 10 HPF and $\geq$20% Ki-67 index). An adeno component may be observed.[23,30,31] Gastric NECs arise in elderly patients, with no sex prevalence, at any part of the stomach, and high stage at diagnosis.[29] Survival is poor, most patients dying within a few months. The *p53* gene is usually abnormal, indicating the substantially diverse genetic background[44,45] as compared with gastrin-dependent NETs. Nonetheless, the progression from G2 NETs to NEC is suggested by some rare cases either in an A-CAG or MEN1/ZES background.[23,42]

DUODENUM

Hyperplasia-dysplasia

A recent systematic study in subjects with MEN1-ZES demonstrated that duodenal gastrin undergo changes similar to those described for gastric nonantral endocrine cells with (**Table 3**).[46] Patterns of diffuse, linear, and micronodular hyperplasia and additional enlarged and microinvasive lesions are detailed. Interestingly, hyperplastic gastrin cell lesions showed a high Ki-67 (proliferative) labeling index. A confirmatory study reported duodenal gastrin cell hyperplasia in 18 subjects with sporadic gastrinomas, *Hp* gastritis, and treated with PPIs (see **Table 3**).[47]

More recently, somatostatin-producing D-cell hyperplasia was demonstrated by a recent analysis of duodenal lesions in patients with MEN1.[48] Because in patients with MEN1 the loss of heterozygosity for 11q13 chromosomal markers at the MEN1 gene locus occurred exclusively in G-cell and D-cell tumor cells but not in hyperplastic lesions, a different genetic mechanism was postulated as the basis of hyperplastic lesions. Thus far, no hyperplastic/dysplastic changes have been described with other types of endocrine cells of the duodenum, despite their abundance in the normal state[49] and their occasional involvement in tumor growth.[50]

Neoplasia

Tumor type

Four different tumor types are observed depending on tumor-cell components and differentiation. G-cell NETs, either functioning (ie, associated with ZES) and nonfunctioning, represent the largest fraction (>60%) and are mainly located in the I and II part of the duodenum (95% of cases).[22] The second most common tumor type is the somatostatin-producing D-cell NET (21%), usually arising in the periampullary region. The third most relevant and frequent tumor type is the gangliocytic paraganglioma (GCP, 9%) mainly located in the periampullary area. The remaining minority of duodenal tumors comprise the exceedingly rare pancreatic polypeptide (PP), EC-cell NETs, undefined differentiated neoplasms, and the rare but lethal high-grade NEC, located in the first 2 parts of the duodenum (see **Table 2**).[22]

Histology and grading

Duodenal NETs show distinct morphologic features according to the cell type they are made of. G-cell NETs display a classic trabecular to gyriform pattern (Soga and Tazawa B type) (**Fig. 2**B).[51] D-cell NETs display a tubular-glandular structure, approximately 60% with psammoma bodies (see **Fig. 2**C). GCP display a typical lobular structure with triphasic differentiation, and with epithelial, fused, and ganglionlike cells.[50,52] High-grade NECs display the usual solid or trabecular growth pattern with areas of necrosis, elevated mitotic count, and Ki-67 index. According to the ENETS grading system, G- and D-cell NETs may span from G1 (nonfunctioning G-cell NETs) to G2, as usually observed in D-cell and functioning G-cell NETs.[46,53] High-grade NECs are G3.

Clinical setting

Duodenal neuroendocrine neoplasms represent up to 22% of gastrointestinal neuroendocrine neoplasms.[54] The male to female ratio is 1.5:1.0, arising in patients of 50–70 years.[55] G-cell tumors are usually small (<1 cm, mean 0.8 cm), submucosal, polypoid lesions, only rarely infiltrative and are greater than 1 cm in size.[55] When functioning, they associate with the ZES (15%–23% of cases) and are often multiple (13%) in patients with MEN1.[56] Usually MEN1-ZES associate with duodenal more than pancreatic G-cell NETs and arise in younger patients keen to develop local lymph node metastases.[22] Nonfunctioning G-cell NETs are usually incidental findings at microscopic examination of gastrectomy samples. Metastases to local lymph nodes

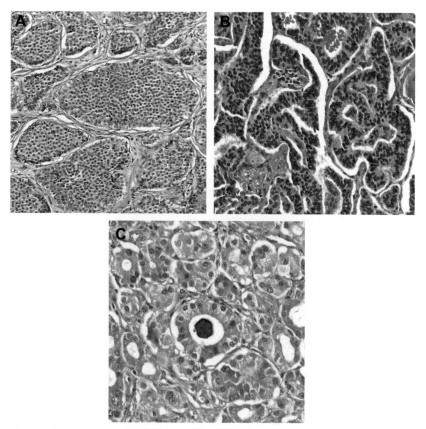

Fig. 2. Histology of gastrointestinal neuroendocrine tumors (NET). (*A*) Typical solid islet structure of a serotonin-producing EC cell NET of the ileum. (*B*) Typical trabecular structure of gastrin-producing G cell NET of the duodenum. (*C*) Typical glandular structure of a somatostatin-producing D cell NET of the duodenum, note the psammoma bodies; hematoxylin and eosin. (*C: Courtesy of* Dr Laura H. Tang, Department of Pathology, Memorial Sloan-Kettering Cancer Center, New York, NY.)

are frequently observed (60%–80%) when associated with ZES and are virtually absent in nonfunctioning cases.[57,58] Their overall survival at 10 years is 60% to 84%.[59]

Larger duodenal neoplasms (see later discussion) may cause either pain, hemorrhage, or obstructive symptoms, including jaundice and pancreatitis. Of the other tumor types, D-cell NETs are usually large (mean size 2.3 cm), deeply infiltrative, and often malignant with metastases. Their overall survival is lower than that observed in G-cell NETs.[22] GCP are large (mean size 1.7 cm), located deeply within the ampullary wall, and are considered as mainly benign.[52] NECs are highly malignant larger masses (2.5 cm) with frequent metastases in the liver and brain.[22] A total of 64% of patients die within 4 to 30 months with a mean survival of 14.5 months.[60]

ILEUM, APPENDIX, AND COLON RECTUM
Hyperplasia Dysplasia

Despite the high frequency of endocrine tumors in the ileum, appendix, and rectum, hyperplastic changes of endocrine cells are rare and reported mainly in association with well-differentiated neuroendocrine (carcinoid) tumors.[61,62] Multiple carcinoid tumors and endocrine cell hyperplasia have been reported in ulcerative colitis and Crohn disease, suggesting chronic, long-standing inflammation may represent a stimulus for endocrine cell growth.[63–66] In these conditions, the proliferating cells are usually argentaffin positive, serotonin-producing, EC cells. It is unknown whether other endocrine cell types participate in this process. Endocrine cell dysplasia has not been reported or defined in these locations. Overall, nonneoplastic proliferative changes of the distal small intestine, appendix, and colon rectum have not been systematically defined.

Neoplasia

Tumor type

The largest fraction of the neuroendocrine neoplasms of the ileum, appendix, and colon rectum are well-differentiated serotonin-producing EC-cell NETs followed by the proglucagon/peptide YY-producing L-cell NETs. As a rule L-cell NETs are observed more often in the large intestine, occasionally found in the appendix and almost absent in the ileum.[67] High-grade NECs are exceedingly rare in the ileum and appendix (only 2 cases reported thus far)[68,69] whereas, they may be observed in the large intestine, often in association with conventional cancer (either adenoma/adenocarcinomas or squamous cell carcinoma in the anal canal).[70]

Histology and grading

EC-cell NETs are characterized by solid islets, with peripheral palisades and occasional glandular aspects (Soga and Tazawa Type A and C structures, respectively) (see **Fig. 2**A).[51] Necrosis is normally absent in both cases. Vessels nearby EC-cell NETs often display a thickened wall with reduced or obstructed lumen.[71] EC-cell NETs display strong argyrophil or argentaffin reactions, strong immunoreactivity for chromogranin A and synaptophysin, as well as for the specific hormones usually stored in EC cells (5HT, substance P, neurokinin A, B and neuropeptide K). Production of growth factors, such as TGF-α, PDGF, αFGF, HGF, TGF-β1 and CTGF, has been described in EC-cell NETs, providing ground for the desmoplastic reaction reported in the mesentery, the vasculature, and the consequently observed symptoms.[72,73]

Conversely, L-cell NETs display a typical trabecular/gyriform pattern (Soga and Tazawa Type B structure). L-cell NETs display immunoreactivity for synaptophysin, for enteroglucagon fragments, including glycentin, GLP1 and GLP2 (GLI1) and pro PP-derived peptides, including peptide YY. Reduced/absent chromogranin A immunoreactivity may be observed in L-cell NETs, likely because of different chromogranin A processing and storage. Expression of the somatostatin receptor subtype 2 (SSR2A) as well as of the transcription factor CDX2 is reported in EC- and L-cell NETs.[74,75] Both EC- and L-cell NETs display only rare mitoses with a Ki-67 index usually at 1% to 2% G1, according to the current grading.[76] High-grade NECs display the morphology similarly observed at other sites, with large areas of necrosis and frequent large-cell aspects (see **Fig. 1**A), small-cell carcinomas more often found in the canal anal.[77]

Clinical settings

The main clinical aspects vary according to the anatomic site. In the ileum the incidence of neuroendocrine neoplasms is 0.28 to 0.89/100,000 per year, accounting for 23% to 28% of all gastrointestinal NET.[78] There is an incidence increase of ileal versus appendiceal NETs and ileal adenocarcinomas or lymphomas.[79] The distribution between sex is equal (male/female ratio of 1:1), involving patients belonging to the VI and VII decades.[22] There is no known genetic defect that associates with ileal neuroendocrine neoplasms; however, high incidence of 18q abnormality is reported.[80,81] MEN1 association is rarely reported for jejunum neoplasms only.[82] Notably, 15% of cases associated with other cancers, mainly adenocarcinomas of the colon. Tumor-specific symptoms are usually absent, including abdominal pain caused by intermittent obstruction and, rarely, melena.[83] The tumor lesions are usually detected by ultrasound, computerized tomography (CT), or video-capsule endoscopy. When liver metastases occur, 5% to 7% develop the carcinoid syndrome.[83,84] Ileal tumors are most frequently greater than or equal to 2 cm (47%) and less than 1 cm in 13%.[85] Nonetheless, deep wall invasion with serosa involvement is frequently observed. When involvement of mesentery occurs, it associates with desmoplasia, intestinal kneeling, and obstruction, rendering reason for the obstructive symptoms most usually observed. The mortality for ileal NETs is 21% versus 6% for the stomach and 4% for the duodenum, with 60% survival at 5 years and 43% at 10 years. Metastatic deposits usually involve mesenteric lymph nodes and liver, but rarely (0.5%) involve other sites. Survival correlates to distance metastases, liver burden, and presence of syndrome.

In the appendix, NETs (carcinoids) represent 50% to 70% of all neoplasms, accounting for 19% of all gastrointestinal NETs.[86] Appendiceal NETs are found in 0.3 to 0.9 of patients with appendectomy, the overall incidence being 0.15/100,000.0 per year.[87,88] Women are more often affected than men in the IV to V decades.[89] Most frequently are asymptomatic, incidental findings located at the tip of the appendix.[90] More rarely, NETs may induce inflammation and appendicitis following lumen obstruction when located at other parts of the organ. Most cases (75%) are located at the tip, 15% are located in the mid portion, and 10% at the base. Usually small, appendiceal NETs are less than 1 cm in size in 80% of cases, 1 to 2 cm in 14%, and greater than 2 cm in 6%.[91] The NET size is the major determinant for the risk of developing metastases, with no metastases observed in lesions less than 1 cm in size, less than 1% risk in 1- to 2-cm lesions, and 21% to 44% risk in tumors greater than 2 cm in size.[89] The survival at 5 years is 88% to 94% for localized NETs, 78% to 83% when associated with regional metastases, and of 25% to 31% in presence of distant metastases.[88]

In the colon rectum, neuroendocrine neoplasms represent 0.4% of all types of colorectal neoplasms.[92] A total of 8% of all gastrointestinal NETs are found in the cecum transverse and 27% are found in the descending colon and rectum, accounting for 0.11 to 0.21/100,000 of new cases per year for the whole large intestine.[93] It is described a descending prevalence of Asian, African, and Native American patients.[92] The observed sex distribution displays a slight male prevalence in the rectum (male/female ratio of 1.02) and a slight female prevalence in the colon (male/female ratio 0.6).[70,93] Usually patients are affected by NETs at a younger age in the rectum (60–70 years) than in the colon (70–80 years).

Colon-rectal NETs are mostly found in the rectum (54%), followed by cecum (20%), sigmoid colon (7.5%), rectum-sigmoid (5.5%), and ascending colon (5%).[93] The reported average size for right-colon NETs is 4.9 cm; whereas, 50% of rectal NETs are less than 1 cm in size, with only 13% greater than 2 cm.[94,95] Only less than 5% of cases develop a carcinoid syndrome; whereas, 50% are asymptomatic.[96] When symptoms are observed they are usually abdominal pain and weight loss and associate with tumor spread.[97] The observed 5-year survival is 25% to 42% for localized disease and 10% for 10 years (Surveillance Epidemiology End Results [SEER], data).[93] However, the 5-year survival for rectal NETs is 72% to 89%.[93,98]

PDECs represent 0.6% of large-bowel carcinoma, and affect mostly the VII decade of patients in both sexes.[70] Symptoms are caused by local or widespread metastases. The most frequent site is the right colon or rectum-sigmoid, with a macroscopic aspect indistinguishable from conventional adenocarcinoma. Local lymph-node spread is observed in 36% to 44% of cases and distant metastases in 38% of cases. High-grade NECs show a morphology similar to that observed for NECs in other sites. However, 75% are composed by large cells (see **Fig. 1**B) in the colon rectum and are often associated with adenomas; whereas, by small cells in the anal canal and often associated with squamous components.[77] Similar to high-grade NECs at other gastrointestinal sites, colorectal NECs are highly aggressive, presenting with metastases at 70% of cases, with a median survival of 10.4 months, a 2-year survival in 25% of cases, and a 5-year survival in 13%.[70,77,99]

REFERENCES

1. Jensen RT. Consequences of long-term proton pump blockade: insights from studies of patients with gastrinomas. Basic Clin Pharmacol Toxicol 2006; 98(1):4–19.
2. Bordi C, Gabrielli M, Missale G. Pathologic changes of endocrine cells in chronic atrophic gastritis. An ultrastructural study on peroral gastric biopsy specimens. Arch Pathol Lab Med 1978;102(3):129–35.
3. Solcia E, Rindi G, Fiocca R, et al. Distinct patterns of chronic gastritis associated with carcinoid and cancer and their role in tumorigenesis. Yale J Biol Med 1992; 65(6):793–804; [discussion: 827–9].
4. Lamberts R, Creutzfeldt W, Struber HG, et al. Long-term omeprazole therapy in peptic ulcer disease: gastrin, endocrine cell growth, and gastritis. Gastroenterology 1993;104(5):1356–70.
5. Solcia E, Bordi C, Creutzfeldt W, et al. Histopathological classification of nonantral gastric endocrine growths in man. Digestion 1988;41:185–200.
6. Solcia E, Capella C, Sessa F, et al. Gastric carcinoids and related endocrine growths. Digestion 1986;35(Suppl 1):3–22.
7. Bordi C, Cocconi G, Togni R, et al. Gastric endocrine cell proliferation. Association with Zollinger-Ellison syndrome. Arch Pathol 1974;98(4):274–8.
8. Solcia E, Capella C, Buffa R, et al. Identification, ultrastructure and classification of gut endocrine cells and related growths. Invest Cell Pathol 1980;3(1):37–49.
9. Bordi C, Ferrari C, D'Adda T, et al. Ultrastructural characterization of fundic endocrine cell hyperplasia associated with atrophic gastritis and hypergastrinaemia. Virchows Arch A Pathol Anat Histopathol 1986;409(3):335–47.
10. Bordi C, Yu JY, Baggi MT, et al. Gastric carcinoids and their precursor lesions. A histologic and immunohistochemical study of 23 cases. Cancer 1991;67(3): 663–72.
11. Srivastava A, Kamath A, Barry SA, et al. Ghrelin expression in hyperplastic and neoplastic proliferations of the enterochromaffin-like (ECL) cells. Endocr Pathol 2004;15(1):47–54.
12. Creutzfeldt W. The achlorhydria-carcinoid sequence: role of gastrin. Digestion 1988;39(2):61–79.
13. D'Adda T, Corleto V, Pilato FP, et al. Quantitative ultrastructure of endocrine cells of oxyntic mucosa in Zollinger-Ellison syndrome. Correspondence with light microscopic findings. Gastroenterology 1990;99(1):17–26.
14. Bordi C, D'Adda T, Azzoni C, et al. Hypergastrinemia and gastric enterochromaffin-like cells. Am J Surg Pathol 1995;19(Suppl 1):S8–19.
15. Arnold R, Hulst MV, Neuhof CH, et al. Antral gastrin-producing G-cells and somatostatin-producing D-cells in different states of gastric acid secretion. Gut 1982;23(4):285–91.

16. Arnold R, Frank M, Simon B, et al. Adaptation and renewal of the endocrine stomach. Scand J Gastroenterol Suppl 1992;193:20–7.
17. Polak JM, Stagg B, Pearse AG. Two types of Zollinger-Ellison syndrome: immuno-fluorescent, cytochemical and ultrastructural studies of the antral and pancreatic gastrin cells in different clinical states. Gut 1972;13(7):501–12.
18. Keuppens F, Willems G, De Graef J, et al. Antral gastrin cell hyperplasia in patients with peptic ulcer. Ann Surg 1980;191(3):276–81.
19. Friesen SR, Tomita T. Pseudo-Zollinger-Ellison syndrome: hypergastrinemia, hyperchlorhydria without tumor. Ann Surg 1981;194(4):481–93.
20. Annibale B, Bonamico M, Rindi G, et al. Antral gastrin cell hyperfunction in children. A functional and immunocytochemical report. Gastroenterology 1991;101(6): 1547–51.
21. Rindi G, Annibale B, Bonamico M, et al. Helicobacter pylori infection in children with antral gastrin cell hyperfunction. J Pediatr Gastroenterol Nutr 1994;18(2):152–8.
22. Solcia E, Capella C, Fiocca R, et al. Disorders of the endocrine system. In: Ming SC, Goldman H, editors. Pathology of the gastrointestinal tract. Philadelphia: Williams and Wilkins; 1998. p. 295–322.
23. Rindi G, Luinetti O, Cornaggia M, et al. Three subtypes of gastric argyrophil carcinoid and the gastric neuroendocrine carcinoma: a clinicopathologic study. Gastroenterology 1993;104(4):994–1006.
24. Papotti M, Cassoni P, Volante M, et al. Ghrelin-producing endocrine tumors of the stomach and intestine. J Clin Endocrinol Metab 2001;86(10):5052–9.
25. Rindi G, Bordi C, Rappel S, et al. Gastric carcinoids and neuroendocrine carcinomas: pathogenesis, pathology, and behavior. World J Surg 1996;20(2):168–72.
26. Quinonez G, Ragbeer MS, Simon GT. A carcinoid tumor of the stomach with features of a midgut tumor. Arch Pathol Lab Med 1988;112(8):838–41.
27. Tsolakis AV, Portela-Gomes GM, Stridsberg M, et al. Malignant gastric ghrelinoma with hyperghrelinemia. J Clin Endocrinol Metab 2004;89(8):3739–44.
28. Rindi G, Kloppel G, Alhman H, et al. TNM staging of foregut (neuro)endocrine tumors: a consensus proposal including a grading system. Virchows Arch 2006;449(4):395–401.
29. Rindi G, Azzoni C, La Rosa S, et al. ECL cell tumor and poorly differentiated endocrine carcinoma of the stomach: prognostic evaluation by pathological analysis. Gastroenterology 1999;116(3):532–42.
30. Jiang SX, Mikami T, Umezawa A, et al. Gastric large cell neuroendocrine carcinomas: a distinct clinicopathologic entity. Am J Surg Pathol 2006;30(8):945–53.
31. Brenner B, Tang LH, Klimstra DS, et al. Small-cell carcinomas of the gastrointestinal tract: a review. J Clin Oncol 2004;22(13):2730–9.
32. Chiaravalli AM, Klersy C, Tava F, et al. Lower- and higher-grade subtypes of diffuse gastric cancer. Hum Pathol 2009;40(11):1591–9.
33. Solcia E, Klersy C, Mastracci L, et al. A combined histologic and molecular approach identifies three groups of gastric cancer with different prognosis. Virchows Arch 2009;455(3):197–211.
34. Rindi G, Kloppel G, Couvelard A, et al. TNM staging of midgut and hindgut (neuro) endocrine tumors: a consensus proposal including a grading system. Virchows Arch 2007;451(4):757–62.
35. Pape UF, Jann H, Muller-Nordhorn J, et al. Prognostic relevance of a novel TNM classification system for upper gastroenteropancreatic neuroendocrine tumors. Cancer 2008;113(2):256–65.
36. Edge SB, Byrd DR, Compton CC, et al, editors. AJCC cancer staging manual. 7th edition. New York: Springer-Verlag; 2010.

37. Hou W, Schubert ML. Treatment of gastric carcinoids. Curr Treat Options Gastroenterol 2007;10(2):123–33.
38. Ooi A, Ota M, Katsuda S, et al. An unusual case of multiple gastric carcinoids associated with diffuse endocrine cell hyperplasia and parietal cell hypertrophy. Endocr Pathol 1995;6(3):229–37.
39. Abraham SC, Carney JA, Ooi A, et al. Achlorhydria, parietal cell hyperplasia, and multiple gastric carcinoids: a new disorder. Am J Surg Pathol 2005;29(7):969–75.
40. Wangberg B, Grimelius L, Granerus G, et al. The role of gastric resection in the management of multicentric argyrophil gastric carcinoids. Surgery 1990;108(5):851–7.
41. Berna MJ, Annibale B, Marignani M, et al. A prospective study of gastric carcinoids and enterochromaffin-like cell changes in multiple endocrine neoplasia type 1 and Zollinger-Ellison syndrome: identification of risk factors. J Clin Endocrinol Metab 2008;93(5):1582–91.
42. Bordi C, Falchetti A, Azzoni C, et al. Aggressive forms of gastric neuroendocrine tumors in multiple endocrine neoplasia type I. Am J Surg Pathol 1997;21(9):1075–82.
43. Norton JA, Melcher ML, Gibril F, et al. Gastric carcinoid tumors in multiple endocrine neoplasia-1 patients with Zollinger-Ellison syndrome can be symptomatic, demonstrate aggressive growth, and require surgical treatment. Surgery 2004;136(6):1267–74.
44. Pizzi S, Azzoni C, Bassi D, et al. Genetic alterations in poorly differentiated endocrine carcinomas of the gastrointestinal tract. Cancer 2003;98(6):1273–82.
45. Furlan D, Bernasconi B, Uccella S, et al. Allelotypes and fluorescence in situ hybridization profiles of poorly differentiated endocrine carcinomas of different sites. Clin Cancer Res 2005;11(5):1765–75.
46. Anlauf M, Perren A, Meyer CL, et al. Precursor lesions in patients with multiple endocrine neoplasia type 1-associated duodenal gastrinomas. Gastroenterology 2005;128(5):1187–98.
47. Merchant SH, VanderJagt T, Lathrop S, et al. Sporadic duodenal bulb gastrin-cell tumors: association with Helicobacter pylori gastritis and long-term use of proton pump inhibitors. Am J Surg Pathol 2006;30(12):1581–7.
48. Anlauf M, Perren A, Henopp T, et al. Allelic deletion of the MEN1 gene in duodenal gastrin and somatostatin cell neoplasms and their precursor lesions. Gut 2007;56(5):637–44.
49. Rindi G, Leiter AB, Kopin AS, et al. The "normal" endocrine cell of the gut. Changing concepts and new evidences. Ann N Y Acad Sci 2004;1014:1–12.
50. Capella C, Riva C, Rindi G, et al. Endocrine tumors of the duodenum and upper jejunum. A study of 33 cases with clinico-pathological characteristics and hormone content. Hepatogastroenterology 1990;37(2):247–52.
51. Soga J, Tazawa K. Pathologic analysis of carcinoids. Histologic reevaluation of 62 cases. Cancer 1971;28(4):990–8.
52. Capella C, Riva C, Rindi G, et al. Histopathology, hormone products and clinicopathologic profile of endocrine tumours of the upper small intestine. A study of 44 cases. Endocr Pathol 1991;2:91–110.
53. Anlauf M, Garbrecht N, Henopp T, et al. Sporadic versus hereditary gastrinomas of the duodenum and pancreas: distinct clinico-pathological and epidemiological features. World J Gastroenterol 2006;12(34):5440–6.
54. Vinik AI, McLeod MK, Fig LM, et al. Clinical features, diagnosis, and localization of carcinoid tumors and their management. Gastroenterol Clin North Am 1989;18(4):865–96.

55. Burke AP, Sobin LH, Federspiel BH, et al. Carcinoid tumors of the duodenum. A clinicopathologic study of 99 cases. Arch Pathol Lab Med 1990;114(7):700–4.

56. Anlauf M, Enosawa T, Henopp T, et al. Primary lymph node gastrinoma or occult duodenal microgastrinoma with lymph node metastases in a MEN1 patient: the need for a systematic search for the primary tumor. Am J Surg Pathol 2008; 32(7):1101–5.

57. Hofmann JW, Fox PS, Wilson SD. Duodenal wall tumors and the Zollinger-Ellison syndrome. Surgical management. Arch Surg 1973;107(2):334–9.

58. Pipeleers-Marichal M, Somers G, Willems G, et al. Gastrinomas in the duodenums of patients with multiple endocrine neoplasia type 1 and the Zollinger-Ellison syndrome. N Engl J Med 1990;322(11):723–7.

59. Weber HC, Venzon DJ, Lin JT, et al. Determinants of metastatic rate and survival in patients with Zollinger-Ellison syndrome: a prospective long-term study. Gastroenterology 1995;108(6):1637–49.

60. Nassar H, Albores-Saavedra J, Klimstra DS. High-grade neuroendocrine carcinoma of the ampulla of Vater: a clinicopathologic and immunohistochemical analysis of 14 cases. Am J Surg Pathol 2005;29(5):588–94.

61. Cross SS, Hughes AD, Williams GT, et al. Endocrine cell hyperplasia and appendiceal carcinoids. J Pathol 1988;156(4):325–9.

62. Moyana TN, Satkunam N. A comparative immunohistochemical study of jejunoileal and appendiceal carcinoids. Implications for histogenesis and pathogenesis. Cancer 1992;70(5):1081–8.

63. Gledhill A, Hall PA, Cruse JP, et al. Enteroendocrine cell hyperplasia, carcinoid tumours and adenocarcinoma in long-standing ulcerative colitis. Histopathology 1986;10(5):501–8.

64. Hock YL, Scott KW, Grace RH. Mixed adenocarcinoma/carcinoid tumour of large bowel in a patient with Crohn's disease. J Clin Pathol 1993;46(2):183–5.

65. Matsumoto T, Jo Y, Mibu R, et al. Multiple microcarcinoids in a patient with long standing ulcerative colitis. J Clin Pathol 2003;56(12):963–5.

66. Nascimbeni R, Villanacci V, Di Fabio F, et al. Solitary microcarcinoid of the rectal stump in ulcerative colitis. Neuroendocrinology 2005;81(6):400–4.

67. Fiocca R, Rindi G, Capella C, et al. Glucagon, glicentin, proglucagon, PYY, PP and proPP-icosapeptide immunoreactivities of rectal carcinoid tumors and related non-tumor cells. Regul Pept 1987;17(1):9–29.

68. O'Kane AM, O'Donnell ME, Shah R, et al. Small cell carcinoma of the appendix. World J Surg Oncol 2008;6:4.

69. Rossi G, Bertolini F, Sartori G, et al. Primary mixed adenocarcinoma and small cell carcinoma of the appendix: a clinicopathologic, immunohistochemical, and molecular study of a hitherto unreported tumor. Am J Surg Pathol 2004;28(9):1233–9.

70. Bernick PE, Klimstra DS, Shia J, et al. Neuroendocrine carcinomas of the colon and rectum. Dis Colon Rectum 2004;47(2):163–9.

71. Anthony PP, Drury RA. Elastic vascular sclerosis of mesenteric blood vessels in argentaffin carcinoma. J Clin Pathol 1970;23(2):110–8.

72. La Rosa S, Chiaravalli AM, Capella C, et al. Immunohistochemical localization of acidic fibroblast growth factor in normal human enterochromaffin cells and related gastrointestinal tumours. Virchows Arch 1997;430(2):117–24.

73. Nilsson O, Wangberg B, McRae A, et al. Growth factors and carcinoid tumours. Acta Oncol 1993;32(2):115–24.

74. Papotti M, Bongiovanni M, Volante M, et al. Expression of somatostatin receptor types 1-5 in 81 cases of gastrointestinal and pancreatic endocrine tumors.

A correlative immunohistochemical and reverse-transcriptase polymerase chain reaction analysis. Virchows Arch 2002;440(5):461–75.

75. La Rosa S, Rigoli E, Uccella S, et al. CDX2 as a marker of intestinal EC-cells and related well-differentiated endocrine tumors. Virchows Arch 2004;445(3):248–54.

76. Canavese G, Azzoni C, Pizzi S, et al. p27: a potential main inhibitor of cell proliferation in digestive endocrine tumors but not a marker of benign behavior. Hum Pathol 2001;32(10):1094–101.

77. Shia J, Tang LH, Weiser MR, et al. Is nonsmall cell type high-grade neuroendocrine carcinoma of the tubular gastrointestinal tract a distinct disease entity? Am J Surg Pathol 2008;32(5):719–31.

78. Schottenfeld D, Beebe-Dimmer JL, Vigneau FD. The epidemiology and pathogenesis of neoplasia in the small intestine. Ann Epidemiol 2009;19(1): 58–69.

79. Modlin IM, Champaneria MC, Chan AK, et al. A three-decade analysis of 3,911 small intestinal neuroendocrine tumors: the rapid pace of no progress. Am J Gastroenterol 2007;102(7):1464–73.

80. Zhao J, de Krijger RR, Meier D, et al. Genomic alterations in well-differentiated gastrointestinal and bronchial neuroendocrine tumors (carcinoids): marked differences indicating diversity in molecular pathogenesis. Am J Pathol 2000;157(5): 1431–8.

81. Tonnies H, Toliat MR, Ramel C, et al. Analysis of sporadic neuroendocrine tumours of the enteropancreatic system by comparative genomic hybridisation. Gut 2001;48(4):536–41.

82. Moertel CG, Dockerty MB. Familial occurrence of metastasizing carcinoid tumors. Ann Intern Med 1973;78(3):389–90.

83. Moertel CG, Sauer WG, Dockerty MB, et al. Life history of the carcinoid tumor of the small intestine. Cancer 1961;14:901–12.

84. Godwin JD 2nd. Carcinoid tumors. An analysis of 2,837 cases. Cancer 1975; 36(2):560–9.

85. Burke AP, Thomas RM, Elsayed AM, et al. Carcinoids of the jejunum and ileum: an immunohistochemical and clinicopathologic study of 167 cases. Cancer 1997; 79(6):1086–93.

86. Lyss AP. Appendiceal malignancies. Semin Oncol 1988;15(2):129–37.

87. Marudanayagam R, Williams GT, Rees BI. Review of the pathological results of 2660 appendicectomy specimens. J Gastroenterol 2006;41(8):745–9.

88. Yao JC, Hassan M, Phan A, et al. One hundred years after "carcinoid": epidemiology of and prognostic factors for neuroendocrine tumors in 35,825 cases in the United States. J Clin Oncol 2008;26(18):3063–72.

89. Moertel CG, Dockerty MB, Judd ES. Carcinoid tumors of the vermiform appendix. Cancer 1968;21(2):270–8.

90. Goede AC, Caplin ME, Winslet MC. Carcinoid tumour of the appendix. Br J Surg 2003;90(11):1317–22.

91. Stinner B, Rothmund M. Neuroendocrine tumours (carcinoids) of the appendix. Best Pract Res Clin Gastroenterol 2005;19(5):729–38.

92. Konishi T, Watanabe T, Kishimoto J, et al. Prognosis and risk factors of metastasis in colorectal carcinoids: results of a nationwide registry over 15 years. Gut 2007; 56(6):863–8.

93. Modlin IM, Sandor A. An analysis of 8305 cases of carcinoid tumors. Cancer 1997;79(4):813–29.

94. Berardi RS. Carcinoid tumors of the colon (exclusive of the rectum): review of the literature. Dis Colon Rectum 1972;15(5):383–91.

95. Kwaan MR, Goldberg JE, Bleday R. Rectal carcinoid tumors: review of results after endoscopic and surgical therapy. Arch Surg 2008;143(5):471–5.
96. Rosenberg JM, Welch JP. Carcinoid tumors of the colon. A study of 72 patients. Am J Surg 1985;149(6):775–9.
97. Stinner B, Kisker O, Zielke A, et al. Surgical management for carcinoid tumors of small bowel, appendix, colon, and rectum. World J Surg 1996; 20(2):183–8.
98. Modlin IM, Lye KD, Kidd MA. 5-decade analysis of 13,715 carcinoid tumors. Cancer 2003;97(4):934–59.
99. Brenner B, Tang LH, Shia J, et al. Small cell carcinomas of the gastrointestinal tract: clinicopathological features and treatment approach. Semin Oncol 2007; 34(1):43–50.

Appetite and Hedonism: Gut Hormones and the Brain

Katherine A. Simpson, MB, ChB, MRCP,
Stephen R. Bloom, MA, MD, DSc, FRCPath, FRCP, FMedSci*

KEYWORDS

- Appetite • Food • Gut hormones • Hypothalamus
- Brainstem • Reward

The ability to maintain adequate food intake is fundamental to survival. At times of famine, the drive to maintain energy intake can be so powerful that humans resort to extreme behavior to survive. For example, it was such a situation that drove the Nantucket crew onboard the Essex whaleship in 1820 to break all taboos and resort to cannibalism in their lifeboat after the ship was sunk by a sperm whale.[1] In contrast, when homeostatic mechanisms controlling food intake are poorly adapted to the unique modern environment of plenty, both excess energy intake and reduced exercise result in widespread obesity. Globally, the World Health Organization (WHO) estimates that more than 1 billion adults and more than 42 million children younger than 5 years are overweight.[2,3] Obesity is associated with diabetes mellitus, hyperlipidemia, hypertension, cardiovascular disease, and certain forms of cancer.[4] Evolutionarily, it is advantageous that the consumption of food is associated with feelings of reward, and at times of famine the stored energy is utilized efficiently when needed. However, in today's society, such reward-seeking behavior and the constant availability of highly palatable food is a major factor for the increased incidence of obesity.

The control of food intake is complex and consists of neural and hormonal signals between the gut and central nervous system (CNS). In addition, signals relating to energy reserves such as adipose tissue, as well as genetic predisposition to obesity, are involved. The brain is responsible for interpreting the signals from the periphery and increasing or decreasing food intake depending on energy reserves and the wanting of food. Even before eating, gut hormones are released and begin the process of meal termination and feelings of satiation. Gut hormones act within key brain areas

Section of Investigative Medicine, Imperial College London, Commonwealth Building, Du Cane Road, London, W12 0NN, UK
* Corresponding author.
E-mail address: s.bloom@imperial.ac.uk

Endocrinol Metab Clin N Am 39 (2010) 729–743
doi:10.1016/j.ecl.2010.08.001

such as the hypothalamus and brainstem, which contain intricate neuronal networks and connections to other parts of the brain that are involved with reward and desirability.

As such, there is a basic need for centers within the brain to be able to respond at times of hunger or satiation and adjust food intake accordingly. However, reward centers can override this mechanism beyond homeostatic need when faced with desirable and palatable food.

HYPOTHALAMUS

The hypothalamus consists of several important nuclei that are involved in appetite control and energy homeostasis: the arcuate nucleus (ARCN), paraventricular nucleus (PVN), ventromedial nucleus (VMN), dorsomedial nucleus (DMN), and lateral hypothalamic area (LHA). These nuclei receive neuronal connections from other parts of the brain, such as the brain stem (which receives gut vagal afferents) and reward centers (**Fig. 1**). In addition, certain hormones such as insulin and leptin are able to exert a direct effect via the circulation and access the ARCN via a saturable process across the blood-brain barrier (BBB). Some investigators have postulated that there is also an incomplete BBB at the median eminence of the hypothalamus and area postrema of the brainstem, perhaps allowing other peptides to act directly on important CNS centers that control food intake.

Arcuate Nucleus

The ARCN contains many neuronal populations involved in food intake. Of these, the best characterized are the neuropeptide Y (NPY)/agouti-related protein (AgRP) neurons, which increase food intake (orexigenic),[5–9] and the cocaine- and amphetamine-regulated transcript (CART)/proopiomelanocortin (POMC) neurons which inhibit food intake (anorexigenic).[10,11] Both populations receive signals from the periphery via the circulation and brainstem projections. In addition, arcuate neurones have extensive projections within the hypothalamus, including the PVN, DMN, and LHA.[12–14] Among the POMC neurons, alpha-melanocyte-stimulating hormone (α-MSH) binds to the melanocortin (MC) receptor 4 in the PVN.[15] AgRP is coexpressed with NPY in the ARCN and is an endogenous antagonist at the MC3 and MC4 receptors.[8] In humans, MC4 receptor mutations account for approximately 6% of severe early-onset obesity, and as many as 90 different MC4 receptor mutations have been associated with obesity.[16,17] MC4 receptors are also found in the brainstem, where overexpression of α-MSH causes a reduction in food intake and weight loss.[18] Receptors are also found in the amygdala and lateral hypothalamus, which form part of the mesolimbic reward system. CART is a neurotransmitter that appears to have different effects depending on the site of administration. Injection into the third ventricle inhibits food intake,[19,20] whereas injection into hypothalamic nuclei such as the VMN, ARCN, or PVN causes an increase in food intake and obesity.[20]

Paraventricular Nucleus

NPY/AgRP and CART/POMC neurons from the ARCN project to the PVN neurons containing corticotropin-releasing hormone (CRH) and thyrotropin-releasing hormone (TRH),[21–23] both of which are involved in the modulation of food intake and energy expenditure.[24–26] Chronic NPY overexpression in the PVN results in hyperphagia and obesity in rats.[27] CRH is an anorexigenic neuropeptide, and messenger RNA (mRNA) levels in the PVN decrease during starvation.[25] TSH acts centrally to reduce food intake, and during fasting, TRH gene expression is downregulated in the PVN.[26]

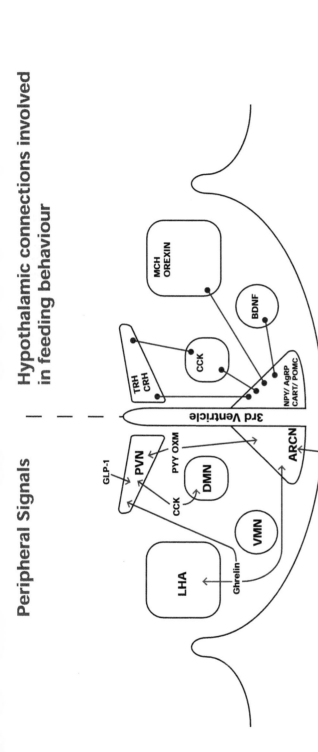

Fig. 1. Peripheral signals acting within key hypothalamic nuclei on the left of the dotted line. To the right, major signaling pathways and neuronal networks implicated in feeding control. BDNF, brain-derived neurotrophic factor; CCK, cholecystokinin; CRH, corticotropin-releasing hormone; GLP-1, glucagon-like peptide 1; MCH, melanin concentrating hormone; OXM, oxyntomodulin; PYY, peptide tyrosine tyrosine; TRH, thyrotrophin-releasing hormone.

Dorsomedial Nucleus

Lesioning of the DMN results in hyperphagia and obesity.[28] The DMN contains a large number of NPY and α-MSH terminals originating from the ARCN.[29,30] Overexpression of NPY in the DMN increases food intake and body weight.[31] Cholecystokinin (CCK) 1 receptors and NPY colocalize within the DMN. Administration of CCK into the DMN downregulates NPY gene expression and inhibits food intake in rats.[32] In addition, CCK1 knockout rats are hyperphagic and demonstrate an increased NPY mRNA expression in the DMN.[33] α-MSH fibers also project from the DMN to the PVN, terminating on TRH-expressing neurons.[34]

Ventromedial Nucleus

The VMN is largely involved with glucose homeostasis. The VMN receives NPY, AgRP, and POMC neuronal projections from the ARCN. The MC4 receptor is highly expressed in the VMN, and direct injection of α-MSH causes a significant increase in feeding.[35] It is thought that brain-derived neurotrophic factor (BDNF) is a downstream effector for the melanocortin-induced anorexia, and disruption of BDNF signaling in the brainstem, VMN, DMN, and PVN has been implicated in the control of feeding behavior.[36,37]

Lateral Hypothalamus

NPY, AgRP, and α-MSH immunoreactive terminals are extensive in the LHA and terminate on orexigenic melanin-concentrating hormone (MCH) and orexin-expressing cells.[38] MCH immunoreactive fibers also project to the cortex and brainstem. MCH-R1 knockout mice and MCH null mice have increased energy expenditure and are resistant to diet-induced obesity.[39,40] Fasting increases the expression of MCH mRNA, and injection of MCH into the lateral ventricle of rats increases food intake.[41] Central administration of orexins increases food intake[42]; however, subsequent studies proposed that this effect may reflect associated heightened arousal and reduced sleep.[43]

GUT HORMONES

The gastrointestinal tract is the body's largest endocrine organ and produces more than 100 peptides. Anticipation of a meal, mechanical stimulation caused by the presence of food in the stomach, and gut nutrient content result in the secretion of gut hormones, which initiate or terminate food consumption. **Fig. 2** shows the main gut hormones involved in the regulation of food intake.

Peptide Tyrosine Tyrosine

Peptide tyrosine tyrosine (PYY) is a member of the pancreatic polypeptide (PP) fold family of peptides released by L-cells in the gut into the circulation after a meal. Members of the PP-fold family include NPY, PYY, and PP, which share a common tertiary structure called the PP-fold and are involved in food intake regulation. PYY is a 36 amino-acid peptide,which is cleaved at the N-terminus by dipeptidyl peptidase IV (DPP-IV) to create the truncated form, PYY_{3-36}. Full-length PYY binds to the G-protein–coupled receptors Y1, Y2, and Y5. PYY_{3-36} has the highest affinity for the Y2 receptor and is able to cross the BBB freely by a nonsaturable mechanism.[44] The Y2 receptor is an inhibitory presynaptic receptor that is highly expressed on arcuate NPY neurons.[45] NPY neurons also release γ-aminobutyric acid (GABA), which causes tonic inhibition of POMC neurons.[7] Therefore, the anorectic action of PYY

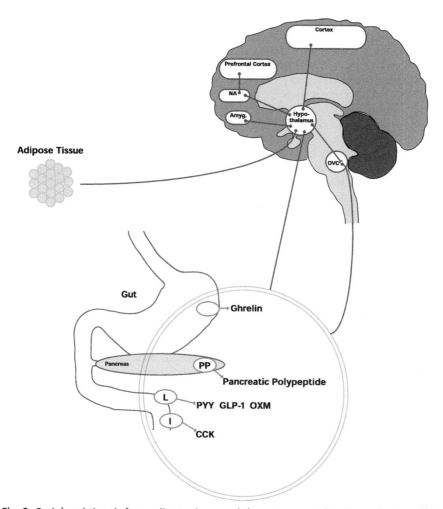

Fig. 2. Peripheral signals from adipose tissue and the gut can act directly on the hypothalamus or via vagal afferents to the brainstem. There are neuronal projections between the brainstem, hypothalamus, cortex, and reward centers in the brain, all of which regulate food intake and energy expenditure. amyg, amygdala; DVC, dorsal vagal complex; GLP-1, glucagon-like peptide 1; NA, nucleus accumbens; OXM, oxyntomodulin; PP, pancreatic polypeptide; PYY, peptide tyrosine tyrosine.

occurs through inhibition of NPY neurons and reduction of GABA-mediated inhibition of POMC neurons.

PYY is released into the circulation after a meal, with levels rising to a plateau after 1 to 2 hours and remaining elevated for up to 6 hours.[46] The increase in PYY levels is proportional to caloric intake and meal composition, so that fatty meals result in a higher increase compared with protein or carbohydrate meals.[47] PYY_{3-36} reduces food intake and body weight in rodents and humans[48,49] and improves insulin sensitivity in rodent models of diet-induced obesity.[50] In obese subjects, the increase in PYY after a meal is blunted, resulting in impaired satiety and hence greater food intake.[51]

After a meal, the anorectic effects of PYY_{3-36} are thought to be predominantly mediated through the Y2 receptors in the ARCN. Peripheral administration of PYY_{3-36} induces c-fos expression (a marker of neuronal activation) in the ARCN, and direct injection of PYY_{3-36} into the ARCN inhibits feeding.[48] This effect is abolished in Y2 receptor knockout mice[48] and after intra-arcuate injection of the Y2 receptor antagonist, B11E0246, in normal mice.[52]

In addition to the hypothalamic effect of PYY_{3-36}, there is evidence that PYY_{3-36} also acts at the brainstem. Y2 receptors are found in important brainstem regions that are involved with appetite control, such as the area postrema and nucleus tractus solitarius.[53,54] Peripheral administration of PYY_{3-36} causes c-fos activation in these areas,[55] and lesioning of the brainstem-hypothalamic neuronal pathways or vagotomy abolishes the anorectic effects of peripheral PYY_{3-36}[53,56] It therefore seems that PYY_{3-36} can also exert an anorectic affect via the vagus nerve to the brainstem, which in turn has connections to the hypothalamus.

Pancreatic Polypeptide

PP is secreted by the PP cells in the pancreatic islets of Langerhans after a meal, and the amount secreted is proportional to the number of calories ingested. Peripheral injection of PP in mice, dogs, and humans causes a dose-dependent reduction in food intake.[57–59] Transgenic mice that overexpress PP are lean and demonstrate reduced food intake.[60] In human studies, intravenous infusion of PP causes a significant reduction in hunger and food intake on presentation of a buffet meal.[61] The anorectic effects are thought to be principally mediated through the Y4 receptor, because the effect is abolished in Y4 receptor knockout mice.[62] Intraperitoneal administration of PP causes c-fos activation in the area postrema and nucleus tractus solitarius (NTS) of the brainstem and in the ARCN, PVN, DMN, VMN, and LHA of the hypothalamus.[63] Y4 receptors are highly expressed in all these regions.[64]

Glucagon-Like Peptide 1

Glucagon-like peptide (GLP)-1, GLP-2, oxyntomodulin (OXM), and glucagon are peptides derived from proglucagon. GLP-1 is cosecreted with PYY from L-cells of the small intestine after a meal.[65] Recent evidence also suggests that GLP-1 is secreted before a meal, also known as a cephalic response to food anticipation.[66] A similar response is seen with insulin and PP and is thought to prepare an animal for the meal and the ensuing nutrient load. GLP-1 exerts its anorectic effect through the activation of the GLP-1 receptor and stimulation of adenylyl cyclase. Peripheral administration of GLP-1 reduces food intake, suppresses glucagon secretion, and delays gastric emptying.[67] Animal studies have shown that peripherally administered GLP-1 induces c-fos expression in the NTS and area postrema of the brainstem,[68] amygdala,[68] and PVN of the hypothalamus.[69,70] Vagotomy or ablation of the brainstem-hypothalamic pathways attenuates the anorectic effect of GLP-1.[56]

GLP-1 also has a potent incretin effect and stimulates insulin in a glucose-dependent manner. Because of the degradation by DPP-IV, however, the half-life is just 1 to 2 minutes.[71] GLP-1 analogues, such as exenatide and liraglutide, are resistant to DPP-IV degradation and are currently licensed for use in patients with type 2 diabetes. Studies show that GLP-1 analogues not only improve glycated hemoglobin A_{1c} levels but also cause weight loss.[72,73]

Oxyntomodulin

As with GLP-1, OXM is secreted by the intestinal L-cells after a meal. Administration of OXM reduces food intake and increases energy expenditure in rodents and humans.[74,75] Although no true receptor has been identified for OXM, the GLP-1 receptor seems to be implicated because the GLP-1 receptor antagonist exending-39 blocks the anorectic effect of OXM.[69,75] In addition, the effect of OXM on food intake is not found in GLP-1 receptor knockout mice.[69] However, manganese-enhanced magnetic resonance imaging in mice demonstrates a difference in the brain region signal in response to GLP-1 or OXM, thereby suggesting that GLP-1 and OXM act via different pathways within the brain to affect food intake.[76]

Cholecystokinin

CCK was the first gut hormone shown to have an effect on food intake.[77] CCK is released from the I-cell of the small intestine, and levels increase rapidly after a meal, reaching a peak within 15 minutes.[78] Peripheral administration of CCK reduces food intake in rodents and humans.[77,79] Although there are 2 CCK receptors, CCK1 and CCK2, the anorectic effect seems to be mediated through the CCK1 receptor. CCK1 receptor knockout rats are obese, and intraperitoneal injection of a CCK1 antagonist results in weight gain.[80,81] However, results of feeding studies to date have been conflicting, and although CCK infusions in rodents decreases meal size, some reports have found a compensatory increase in meal frequency.[82]

Intraperitoneal administration of CCK increases c-fos expression in the DMN and CART neurons in the PVN.[83,84] Direct administration of CCK into the DMN decreases food intake[85] and downregulates NPY gene expression.[80,86] The anorectic effect of CCK is abolished after vagotomy,[87] suggesting that vagal afferent fibers signaling to the dorsal vagal complex in the brainstem are responsible for the reduction in food intake.[88]

Ghrelin

Unlike other gut hormones, ghrelin initiates hunger before a meal and increases food intake.[89,90] Ghrelin is produced by the stomach and is an endogenous ligand for the growth hormone secretagogue receptor. Ghrelin immunoreactive neurons are found adjacent to the third ventricle in the brain and between the DMN, VMN, PVN, and ARCN in the hypothalamus. Furthermore, ghrelin neurons have terminals on the hypothalamic NPY/AgRP, POMC, and CRH neurons in addition to the orexin fibers in the LHA.[91–93] It seems that the orexigenic effect of ghrelin is mediated predominantly through NPY/AgRP arcuate neurons. Peripheral administration of ghrelin stimulates c-fos expression in ARCN NPY/AgRP neurons and increases hypothalamic NPY mRNA expression.[89] Ghrelin-induced feeding is abolished by the central administration of NPY and AgRP antibodies and antagonists in rats[89] and in NPY and AgRP null mice.[94]

In addition to the effects on arcuate NPY/AgRP neurons, intraperitoneal administration of ghrelin also stimulates c-fos expression in the PVN.[95] Direct injection of ghrelin into the PVN stimulates food intake, whereas pretreatment of the intra-PVN injection with a melanocortin agonist suppresses this effect.[96] The effect is also suppressed after the subcutaneous administration of rimonabant, an endocannabinoid CB1 receptor antagonist,[97] and ghrelin does not induce an orexigenic effect in CB1 receptor knockout mice.[98]

ADIPOSITY SIGNALS

Leptin is secreted by adipocytes and circulates at concentrations proportional to the fat mass. Leptin administration decreases food intake and body weight; however, large amounts of adipose tissue, resulting in high circulating levels of leptin, lead to leptin resistance and a lack of the expected anorectic effect. Rodents and humans lacking leptin (ob/ob mice) or the leptin receptor (db/db mice) are obese and hyperphagic; however, this condition can be ameliorated by leptin administration. Leptin is able to cross the BBB and bind to the leptin receptor (Ob-Rb) in the hypothalamus.[99] The predominant effects of leptin on food intake and energy expenditure are mediated in the ARCN, PVN, and LHA. In the ARCN, leptin activates anorectic POMC neurons and inhibits orexigenic AgRP/NPY neurons.[7,100] Leptin also decreases the levels of MCH and orexin and increases CRH gene expression in the hypothalamus,[101–103] and leptin administration seems to modulate ghrelin signaling in the ARCN.[90] In the VMN, inactivation of the leptin receptor results in obesity,[104] and there is now increasing evidence that leptin may affect food intake through actions in the brainstem.[105]

Insulin also acts as an adiposity signal in the brain. Like leptin, insulin can cross the BBB and cause reduced food intake and increased energy expenditure. Insulin inhibits NPY/AgRP neurons in the ARCN. However, the anorectic effects of insulin may also reflect an interaction with the melanocortin system because insulin receptors are also present on the ARCN POMC neurons and intracerebroventricular administration of insulin increases ARCN POMC mRNA expression. Furthermore, the anorectic actions of insulin are blocked by melanocortin antagonists.[106,107]

REWARD PATHWAYS

Reward pathways in the brain involved in feeding behavior include the nucleus accumbens, ventral striatum, ventral tegmental area (VTA), prefrontal cortex, and hippocampus. Conditioned taste aversion and lesioning experiments demonstrate that the orbitofrontal cortex and amygdala are important in learning about and experiencing food. Furthermore, the orbitofrontal cortex receives sensory inputs from the taste, smell, sight, and feel of food in the mouth, as well as chemical composition.[108] Neuroimaging studies in humans have shown that pleasant and unpleasant odors activate different regions of the orbitofrontal cortex and cingulate gyrus.[109] If a meal is eaten to satiety, the signal from the orbitofrontal cortex decreases and the feeding behavior changes from acceptance of food to rejection. This ability to switch from liking food to rejecting food has been associated with leptin signaling. Insulin and leptin receptors are also expressed in these areas,[110] and direct administration of leptin into the VTA decreases food intake in rats.[111] Patients with congenital leptin deficiency are hyperphagic and obese. Leptin treatment not only ameliorates the obesity but also enables patients to discriminate between the "liking ratings" of food in fed and fasted states.[112]

The mesolimbic dopaminergic system is particularly important in feeding behavior. After ingestion of highly palatable food, dopamine levels are increased in the nucleus accumbens.[113] Leptin decreases dopaminergic neuronal firing in ex vivo VTA slices.[114] Ghrelin increases dopamine levels in the nucleus accumbens,[115] and direct injection of ghrelin into the nucleus accumbens and VTA promotes feeding.[116] Endocannabinoids also increase food intake via the cannabinoid CB1 receptor. CB1 receptors are highly expressed in the reward centers and modulate dopaminergic signaling in these regions.[117,118] Blocking CB1 receptors using antagonists, such as rimonabant, inhibits food intake and results in weight loss in rodents and humans.[119,120]

SUMMARY

Obesity is a major worldwide problem, yet unraveling the underlying mechanisms that control food intake and energy homeostasis is complex and evolving. Gut hormones are released in anticipation of a meal and on nutrient load within the gut and signal directly to the hypothalamus or via vagal afferents to the brainstem. The brainstem has projections to the hypothalamus, within which multiple nuclei have onward connections to other regions within the brain that are involved with reward and satiety. As such, the brain is responsible for the integration of these peripheral signals and, based on energy homeostatic need, modulates feeding behavior and thus energy intake. However, it seems that this system can be overridden by reward pathways in the brain, so that the presence of palatable and hence rewarding food, is consumed irrespective of energy requirements.

REFERENCES

1. Philbrick N. In the heart of the sea: the tragedy of the Whaleship Essex. New York: Penguin Books; 2001.
2. Tunstall-Pedoe H. Preventing chronic diseases. A vital investment: World Health Organization. Geneva: World Health Organization; 2005. p. 200.
3. Genomics and World Health, Report of the Advisory Committee on Health Research – Summary. Geneva: World Health Organization; 2002.
4. Must A, Spadano J, Coakley EH, et al. The disease burden associated with overweight and obesity. JAMA 1999;282(16):1523–9.
5. Clark JT, Kalra PS, Crowley WR, et al. Neuropeptide Y and human pancreatic polypeptide stimulate feeding behavior in rats. Endocrinology 1984;115(1): 427–9.
6. Stanley BG, Kyrkouli SE, Lampert S, et al. Neuropeptide Y chronically injected into the hypothalamus: a powerful neurochemical inducer of hyperphagia and obesity. Peptides 1986;7(6):1189–92.
7. Roseberry AG, Liu H, Jackson AC, et al. Neuropeptide Y-mediated inhibition of proopiomelanocortin neurons in the arcuate nucleus shows enhanced desensitization in ob/ob mice. Neuron 2004;41(5):711–22.
8. Ollmann MM, Wilson BD, Yang YK, et al. Antagonism of central melanocortin receptors in vitro and in vivo by agouti-related protein. Science 1997; 278(5335):135–8.
9. Rossi M, Kim MS, Morgan DG, et al. A C-terminal fragment of agouti-related protein increases feeding and antagonizes the effect of alpha-melanocyte stimulating hormone in vivo. Endocrinology 1998;139(10):4428–31.
10. Stanley SA, Small CJ, Murphy KG, et al. Actions of cocaine- and amphetamine-regulated transcript (CART) peptide on regulation of appetite and hypothalamo-pituitary axes in vitro and in vivo in male rats. Brain Res 2001; 893(1–2):186–94.
11. Williams DL, Schwartz MW. The melanocortin system as a central integrator of direct and indirect controls of food intake. Am J Physiol Regul Integr Comp Physiol 2005;289(1):R2–3.
12. Bagnol D, Lu XY, Kaelin CB, et al. Anatomy of an endogenous antagonist: relationship between agouti-related protein and proopiomelanocortin in brain. J Neurosci 1999;19(18):RC26.
13. Broberger C, Johansen J, Johansson C, et al. The neuropeptide Y/agouti gene-related protein (AGRP) brain circuitry in normal, anorectic, and monosodium glutamate-treated mice. Proc Natl Acad Sci U S A 1998;95(25):15043–8.
14. Baker RA, Herkenham M. Arcuate nucleus neurons that project to the hypothalamic paraventricular nucleus: neuropeptidergic identity and consequences of adrenalectomy on mRNA levels in the rat. J Comp Neurol 1995; 358(4):518–30.

15. Cone RD. Studies on the physiological functions of the melanocortin system. Endocr Rev 2006;27(7):736–49.
16. Krude H, Biebermann H, Luck W, et al. Severe early-onset obesity, adrenal insufficiency and red hair pigmentation caused by POMC mutations in humans. Nat Genet 1998;19(2):155–7.
17. Loos RJ, Lindgren CM, Li S, et al. Common variants near MC4R are associated with fat mass, weight and risk of obesity. Nat Genet 2008;40(6):768–75.
18. Li G, Zhang Y, Rodrigues E, et al. Melanocortin activation of nucleus of the solitary tract avoids anorectic tachyphylaxis and induces prolonged weight loss. Am J Physiol Endocrinol Metab 2007;293(1):e252–8.
19. Kristensen P, Judge ME, Thim L, et al. Hypothalamic CART is a new anorectic peptide regulated by leptin. Nature 1998;393(6680):72–6.
20. Abbott CR, Rossi M, Wren AM, et al. Evidence of an orexigenic role for cocaine- and amphetamine-regulated transcript after administration into discrete hypothalamic nuclei. Endocrinology 2001;142(8):3457–63.
21. Fekete C, Legradi G, Mihaly E, et al. Alpha-melanocyte-stimulating hormone is contained in nerve terminals innervating thyrotropin-releasing hormone-synthesizing neurons in the hypothalamic paraventricular nucleus and prevents fasting-induced suppression of prothyrotropin-releasing hormone gene expression. J Neurosci 2000;20(4):1550–8.
22. Legradi G, Lechan RM. Agouti-related protein containing nerve terminals innervate thyrotropin-releasing hormone neurons in the hypothalamic paraventricular nucleus. Endocrinology 1999;140(8):3643–52.
23. Fuzesi T, Wittmann G, Liposits Z, et al. Contribution of noradrenergic and adrenergic cell groups of the brainstem and agouti-related protein-synthesizing neurons of the arcuate nucleus to neuropeptide-Y innervation of corticotropin-releasing hormone neurons in hypothalamic paraventricular nucleus of the rat. Endocrinology 2007;148(11):5442–50.
24. Martin NM, Smith KL, Bloom SR, et al. Interactions between the melanocortin system and the hypothalamo-pituitary-thyroid axis. Peptides 2006;27(2):333–9.
25. Nishiyama M, Makino S, Iwasaki Y, et al. CRH mRNA expression in the hypothalamic paraventricular nucleus is inhibited despite the activation of the hypothalamo-pituitary-adrenal axis during starvation. Brain Res 2008;1228:107–12.
26. Blake NG, Eckland DJ, Foster OJ, et al. Inhibition of hypothalamic thyrotropin-releasing hormone messenger ribonucleic acid during food deprivation. Endocrinology 1991;129(5):2714–8.
27. Tiesjema B, Adan RA, Luijendijk MC, et al. Differential effects of recombinant adeno-associated virus-mediated neuropeptide Y overexpression in the hypothalamic paraventricular nucleus and lateral hypothalamus on feeding behavior. J Neurosci 2007;27(51):14139–46.
28. Bernardis LL, Bellinger LL. The dorsomedial hypothalamic nucleus revisited: 1986 update. Brain Res 1987;434(3):321–81.
29. Chronwall BM, DiMaggio DA, Massari VJ, et al. The anatomy of neuropeptide-Y-containing neurons in rat brain. Neuroscience 1985;15(4):1159–81.
30. Jacobowitz DM, O'Donohue TL. Alpha-melanocyte stimulating hormone: immunohistochemical identification and mapping in neurons of rat brain. Proc Natl Acad Sci U S A 1978;75(12):6300–4.
31. Yang L, Scott KA, Hyun J, et al. Role of dorsomedial hypothalamic neuropeptide Y in modulating food intake and energy balance. J Neurosci 2009;29(1):179–90.
32. Bi S, Scott KA, Kopin AS, et al. Differential roles for cholecystokinin A receptors in energy balance in rats and mice. Endocrinology 2004;145(8):3873–80.

33. Moran TH. Unraveling the obesity of OLETF rats. Physiol Behav 2008;94(1): 71–8.
34. Mihaly E, Fekete C, Legradi G, et al. Hypothalamic dorsomedial nucleus neurons innervate thyrotropin-releasing hormone-synthesizing neurons in the paraventricular nucleus. Brain Res 2001;891(1–2):20–31.
35. Kim MS, Rossi M, Abusnana S, et al. Hypothalamic localization of the feeding effect of agouti-related peptide and alpha-melanocyte-stimulating hormone. Diabetes 2000;49(2):177–82.
36. Bariohay B, Roux J, Tardivel C, et al. Brain-derived neurotrophic factor/tropomy-osin-related kinase receptor type B signaling is a downstream effector of the brainstem melanocortin system in food intake control. Endocrinology 2009; 150(6):2646–53.
37. Xu B, Goulding EH, Zang K, et al. Brain-derived neurotrophic factor regulates energy balance downstream of melanocortin-4 receptor. Nat Neurosci 2003; 6(7):736–42.
38. Broberger C, De LL, Sutcliffe JG, et al. Hypocretin/orexin- and melanin-concen-trating hormone-expressing cells form distinct populations in the rodent lateral hypothalamus: relationship to the neuropeptide Y and agouti gene-related protein systems. J Comp Neurol 1998;402(4):460–74.
39. Chen Y, Hu C, Hsu CK, et al. Targeted disruption of the melanin-concentrating hormone receptor-1 results in hyperphagia and resistance to diet-induced obesity. Endocrinology 2002;143(7):2469–77.
40. Zhou D, Shen Z, Strack AM, et al. Enhanced running wheel activity of both Mch1r- and Pmch-deficient mice. Regul Pept 2005;124(1–3):53–63.
41. Qu D, Ludwig DS, Gammeltoft S, et al. A role for melanin-concentrating hormone in the central regulation of feeding behaviour. Nature 1996; 380(6571):243–7.
42. Sakurai T, Amemiya A, Ishii M, et al. Orexins and orexin receptors: a family of hypothalamic neuropeptides and G protein-coupled receptors that regulate feeding behavior. Cell 1998;92(5):1.
43. Hagan JJ, Leslie RA, Patel S, et al. Orexin A activates locus coeruleus cell firing and increases arousal in the rat. Proc Natl Acad Sci U S A 1999;96(19):10911–6.
44. Nonaka N, Shioda S, Niehoff ML, et al. Characterization of blood-brain barrier permeability to PYY3–36 in the mouse. J Pharmacol Exp Ther 2003;306(3): 948–53.
45. Broberger C, Landry M, Wong H, et al. Subtypes Y1 and Y2 of the neuropeptide Y receptor are respectively expressed in pro-opiomelanocortin- and neuropep-tide-Y-containing neurons of the rat hypothalamic arcuate nucleus. Neuroendo-crinology 1997;66(6):393–408.
46. Adrian TE, Ferri GL, Bacarese-Hamilton AJ, et al. Human distribution and release of a putative new gut hormone, peptide YY. Gastroenterology 1985; 89(5):1070–7.
47. Lin HC, Chey WY. Cholecystokinin and peptide YY are released by fat in either proximal or distal small intestine in dogs. Regul Pept 2003;114(2–3):131–5.
48. Batterham RL, Cowley MA, Small CJ, et al. Gut hormone PYY(3–36) physiolog-ically inhibits food intake. Nature 2002;418(6898):650–4.
49. Batterham RL, Cohen MA, Ellis SM, et al. Inhibition of food intake in obese subjects by peptide YY3–36. N Engl J Med 2003;349(10):941–8.
50. Vrang N, Madsen AN, Tang-Christensen M, et al. PYY(3–36) reduces food intake and body weight and improves insulin sensitivity in rodent models of diet-induced obesity. Am J Physiol Regul Integr Comp Physiol 2006;291(2):R367–75.

51. Le Roux CW, Batterham RL, Aylwin SJ, et al. Attenuated peptide YY release in obese subjects is associated with reduced satiety. Endocrinology 2006;147(1):3–8.

52. Abbott CR, Small CJ, Kennedy AR, et al. Blockade of the neuropeptide Y Y2 receptor with the specific antagonist BIIE0246 attenuates the effect of endogenous and exogenous peptide YY(3–36) on food intake. Brain Res 2005; 1043(1–2):139–44.

53. Koda S, Date Y, Murakami N, et al. The role of the vagal nerve in peripheral PYY3-36-induced feeding reduction in rats. Endocrinology 2005;146(5): 2369–75.

54. Gustafson EL, Smith KE, Durkin MM, et al. Distribution of the neuropeptide Y Y2 receptor mRNA in rat central nervous system. Brain Res Mol Brain Res 1997; 46(1–2):223–35.

55. Blevins JE, Chelikani PK, Haver AC, et al. PYY(3–36) induces Fos in the arcuate nucleus and in both catecholaminergic and non-catecholaminergic neurons in the nucleus tractus solitarius of rats. Peptides 2008;29(1):112–9.

56. Abbott CR, Monteiro M, Small CJ, et al. The inhibitory effects of peripheral administration of peptide YY(3–36) and glucagon-like peptide-1 on food intake are attenuated by ablation of the vagal-brainstem-hypothalamic pathway. Brain Res 2005;1044(1):127–31.

57. Asakawa A, Inui A, Yuzuriha H, et al. Characterization of the effects of pancreatic polypeptide in the regulation of energy balance. Gastroenterology 2003; 124(5):1325–36.

58. Jesudason DR, Monteiro MP, McGowan BM, et al. Low-dose pancreatic polypeptide inhibits food intake in man. Br J Nutr 2007;97(3):426–9.

59. Akerberg H, Meyerson B, Sallander M, et al. Peripheral administration of pancreatic polypeptide inhibits components of food-intake behavior in dogs. Peptides 2010;31(6):1055–61.

60. Ueno N, Inui A, Iwamoto M, et al. Decreased food intake and body weight in pancreatic polypeptide-overexpressing mice. Gastroenterology 1999;117(6): 1427–32.

61. Batterham RL, Le Roux CW, Cohen MA, et al. Pancreatic polypeptide reduces appetite and food intake in humans. J Clin Endocrinol Metab 2003;88(8): 3989–92.

62. Balasubramaniam A, Mullins DE, Lin S, et al. Neuropeptide Y (NPY) Y4 receptor selective agonists based on NPY(32–36): development of an anorectic Y4 receptor selective agonist with picomolar affinity. J Med Chem 2006;49(8): 2661–5.

63. Lin S, Shi YC, Yulyaningsih E, et al. Critical role of arcuate Y4 receptors and the melanocortin system in pancreatic polypeptide-induced reduction in food intake in mice. PLoS One 2009;4(12):e8488.

64. Parker RM, Herzog H. Regional distribution of Y-receptor subtype mRNAs in rat brain. Eur J Neurosci 1999;11(4):1431–48.

65. Ghatei MA, Uttenthal LO, Christofides ND, et al. Molecular forms of human enteroglucagon in tissue and plasma: plasma responses to nutrient stimuli in health and in disorders of the upper gastrointestinal tract. J Clin Endocrinol Metab 1983;57(3):488–95.

66. Williams DL. Expecting to eat: glucagon-like peptide-1 and the anticipation of meals. Endocrinology 2010;151(2):445–7.

67. Verdich C, Flint A, Gutzwiller JP, et al. A meta-analysis of the effect of glucagon-like peptide-1 (7–36) amide on ad libitum energy intake in humans. J Clin Endocrinol Metab 2001;86(9):4382–9.

68. Baumgartner I, Pacheco-Lopez G, Ruttimann EB, et al. Hepatic-portal vein infusions of GLP-1 reduce meal size and increase c-Fos expression in the NTS, AP, and CeA in rats. J Neuroendocrinol 2010;22(6):557–63.
69. Baggio LL, Huang Q, Brown TJ, et al. Oxyntomodulin and glucagon-like peptide-1 differentially regulate murine food intake and energy expenditure. Gastroenterology 2004;127(2):546–58.
70. Dakin CL, Small CJ, Batterham RL, et al. Peripheral oxyntomodulin reduces food intake and body weight gain in rats. Endocrinology 2004;145(6):2687–95.
71. Vilsboll T, Agerso H, Krarup T, et al. Similar elimination rates of glucagon-like peptide-1 in obese type 2 diabetic patients and healthy subjects. J Clin Endocrinol Metab 2003;88(1):220–4.
72. Astrup A, Rossner S, Van GL, et al. Effects of liraglutide in the treatment of obesity: a randomised, double-blind, placebo-controlled study. Lancet 2009; 374(9701):1606–16.
73. Rosenstock J, Klaff LJ, Schwartz S, et al. Effects of exenatide and lifestyle modification on body weight and glucose tolerance in obese subjects with and without prediabetes. Diabetes Care 2010;33(6):1173–5.
74. Wynne K, Park AJ, Small CJ, et al. Oxyntomodulin increases energy expenditure in addition to decreasing energy intake in overweight and obese humans: a randomised controlled trial. Int J Obes (Lond) 2006;30(12):1729–36.
75. Dakin CL, Gunn I, Small CJ, et al. Oxyntomodulin inhibits food intake in the rat. Endocrinology 2001;142(10):4244–50.
76. Chaudhri OB, Parkinson JR, Kuo YT, et al. Differential hypothalamic neuronal activation following peripheral injection of GLP-1 and oxyntomodulin in mice detected by manganese-enhanced magnetic resonance imaging. Biochem Biophys Res Commun 2006;350(2):298–306.
77. Gibbs J, Young RC, Smith GP. Cholecystokinin elicits satiety in rats with open gastric fistulas. Nature 1973;245(5424):323–5.
78. Liddle RA, Goldfine ID, Rosen MS, et al. Cholecystokinin bioactivity in human plasma. Molecular forms, responses to feeding, and relationship to gallbladder contraction. J Clin Invest 1985;75(4):1144–52.
79. Kissileff HR, Pi-Sunyer FX, Thornton J, et al. C-terminal octapeptide of cholecystokinin decreases food intake in man. Am J Clin Nutr 1981;34(2):154–60.
80. Moran TH, Bi S. Hyperphagia and obesity in OLETF rats lacking CCK-1 receptors. Philos Trans R Soc Lond B Biol Sci 2006;361(1471):1211–8.
81. Silver AJ, Flood JF, Song AM, et al. Evidence for a physiological role for CCK in the regulation of food intake in mice. Am J Physiol 1989;256(3 Pt 2):R646–52.
82. West DB, Fey D, Woods SC. Cholecystokinin persistently suppresses meal size but not food intake in free-feeding rats. Am J Physiol 1984;246(5 Pt 2): R776–87.
83. Kobelt P, Paulitsch S, Goebel M, et al. Peripheral injection of CCK-8S induces Fos expression in the dorsomedial hypothalamic nucleus in rats. Brain Res 2006;1117(1):109–17.
84. Peter L, Stengel A, Noetzel S, et al. Peripherally injected CCK-8S activates CART positive neurons of the paraventricular nucleus in rats. Peptides 2010; 31(6):1118–23.
85. Blevins JE, Stanley BG, Reidelberger RD. Brain regions where cholecystokinin suppresses feeding in rats. Brain Res 2000;860(1–2):1–10.
86. Chen J, Scott KA, Zhao Z, et al. Characterization of the feeding inhibition and neural activation produced by dorsomedial hypothalamic cholecystokinin administration. Neuroscience 2008;152(1):178–88.

87. Moran TH, Baldessarini AR, Salorio CF, et al. Vagal afferent and efferent contributions to the inhibition of food intake by cholecystokinin. Am J Physiol 1997; 272(4 Pt 2):R1245–51.

88. Sullivan CN, Raboin SJ, Gulley S, et al. Endogenous cholecystokinin reduces food intake and increases Fos-like immunoreactivity in the dorsal vagal complex but not in the myenteric plexus by CCK1 receptor in the adult rat. Am J Physiol Regul Integr Comp Physiol 2007;292(3):R1071–80.

89. Nakazato M, Murakami N, Date Y, et al. A role for ghrelin in the central regulation of feeding. Nature 2001;409(6817):194–8.

90. Shintani M, Ogawa Y, Ebihara K, et al. Ghrelin, an endogenous growth hormone secretagogue, is a novel orexigenic peptide that antagonizes leptin action through the activation of hypothalamic neuropeptide Y/Y1 receptor pathway. Diabetes 2001;50(2):227–32.

91. Toshinai K, Date Y, Murakami N, et al. Ghrelin-induced food intake is mediated via the orexin pathway. Endocrinology 2003;144(4):1506–12.

92. Willesen MG, Kristensen P, Romer J. Co-localization of growth hormone secretagogue receptor and NPY mRNA in the arcuate nucleus of the rat. Neuroendocrinology 1999;70(5):306–16.

93. Cowley MA, Smith RG, Diano S, et al. The distribution and mechanism of action of ghrelin in the CNS demonstrates a novel hypothalamic circuit regulating energy homeostasis. Neuron 2003;37(4):649–61.

94. Chen HY, Trumbauer ME, Chen AS, et al. Orexigenic action of peripheral ghrelin is mediated by neuropeptide Y and agouti-related protein. Endocrinology 2004; 145(6):2607–12.

95. Ruter J, Kobelt P, Tebbe JJ, et al. Intraperitoneal injection of ghrelin induces Fos expression in the paraventricular nucleus of the hypothalamus in rats. Brain Res 2003;991(1–2):26–33.

96. Shrestha YB, Wickwire K, Giraudo SQ. Action of MT-II on ghrelin-induced feeding in the paraventricular nucleus of the hypothalamus. Neuroreport 2004; 15(8):1365–7.

97. Tucci SA, Rogers EK, Korbonits M, et al. The cannabinoid CB1 receptor antagonist SR141716 blocks the orexigenic effects of intrahypothalamic ghrelin. Br J Pharmacol 2004;143(5):520–3.

98. Kola B, Farkas I, Christ-Crain M, et al. The orexigenic effect of ghrelin is mediated through central activation of the endogenous cannabinoid system. PLoS One 2008;3(3):e1797.

99. Faouzi M, Leshan R, Bjornholm M, et al. Differential accessibility of circulating leptin to individual hypothalamic sites. Endocrinology 2007;148(11):5414–23.

100. Cowley MA, Smart JL, Rubinstein M, et al. Leptin activates anorexigenic POMC neurons through a neural network in the arcuate nucleus. Nature 2001; 411(6836):480–4.

101. Sahu A. Evidence suggesting that galanin (GAL), melanin-concentrating hormone (MCH), neurotensin (NT), proopiomelanocortin (POMC) and neuropeptide Y (NPY) are targets of leptin signaling in the hypothalamus. Endocrinology 1998;139(2):795–8.

102. Lopez M, Seoane L, Garcia MC, et al. Leptin regulation of prepro-orexin and orexin receptor mRNA levels in the hypothalamus. Biochem Biophys Res Commun 2000;269(1):41–5.

103. Huang Q, Rivest R, Richard D. Effects of leptin on corticotropin-releasing factor (CRF) synthesis and CRF neuron activation in the paraventricular hypothalamic nucleus of obese (ob/ob) mice. Endocrinology 1998;139(4):1524–32.

104. Dhillon H, Zigman JM, Ye C, et al. Leptin directly activates SF1 neurons in the VMH, and this action by leptin is required for normal body-weight homeostasis. Neuron 2006;49(2):191–203.

105. Ruiter M, Duffy P, Simasko S, et al. Increased hypothalamic signal transducer and activator of transcription 3 phosphorylation after hindbrain leptin injection. Endocrinology 2010;151(4):1509–19.

106. Kalra SP, Dube MG, Pu S, et al. Interacting appetite-regulating pathways in the hypothalamic regulation of body weight. Endocr Rev 1999;20(1):68–100.

107. Benoit SC, Air EL, Coolen LM, et al. The catabolic action of insulin in the brain is mediated by melanocortins. J Neurosci 2002;22(20):9048–52.

108. Rolls ET. Smell, taste, texture, and temperature multimodal representations in the brain, and their relevance to the control of appetite. Nutr Rev 2004; 62(11 Pt 2):S193–204.

109. Rolls ET. Functions of the orbitofrontal and pregenual cingulate cortex in taste, olfaction, appetite and emotion. Acta Physiol Hung 2008;95(2):131–64.

110. Unger JW, Livingston JN, Moss AM. Insulin receptors in the central nervous system: localization, signalling mechanisms and functional aspects. Prog Neurobiol 1991;36(5):343–62.

111. Morton GJ, Blevins JE, Kim F, et al. The action of leptin in the ventral tegmental area to decrease food intake is dependent on Jak-2 signaling. Am J Physiol Endocrinol Metab 2009;297(1):E202–10.

112. Farooqi IS, Bullmore E, Keogh J, et al. Leptin regulates striatal regions and human eating behavior. Science 2007;317(5843):1355.

113. Hernandez L, Hoebel BG. Food reward and cocaine increase extracellular dopamine in the nucleus accumbens as measured by microdialysis. Life Sci 1988;42(18):1705–12.

114. Hommel JD, Trinko R, Sears RM, et al. Leptin receptor signaling in midbrain dopamine neurons regulates feeding. Neuron 2006;51(6):801–10.

115. Jerlhag E, Egecioglu E, Dickson SL, et al. Ghrelin administration into tegmental areas stimulates locomotor activity and increases extracellular concentration of dopamine in the nucleus accumbens. Addict Biol 2007;12(1):6–16.

116. Naleid AM, Grace MK, Cummings DE, et al. Ghrelin induces feeding in the mesolimbic reward pathway between the ventral tegmental area and the nucleus accumbens. Peptides 2005;26(11):2274–9.

117. Andre VM, Cepeda C, Cummings DM, et al. Dopamine modulation of excitatory currents in the striatum is dictated by the expression of D1 or D2 receptors and modified by endocannabinoids. Eur J Neurosci 2010;31(1):14–28.

118. Sperlagh B, Windisch K, Ando RD, et al. Neurochemical evidence that stimulation of CB1 cannabinoid receptors on GABAergic nerve terminals activates the dopaminergic reward system by increasing dopamine release in the rat nucleus accumbens. Neurochem Int 2009;54(7):452–7.

119. Hildebrandt AL, Kelly-Sullivan DM, Black SC. Antiobesity effects of chronic cannabinoid CB1 receptor antagonist treatment in diet-induced obese mice. Eur J Pharmacol 2003;462(1–3):125–32.

120. Van Gaal LF, Rissanen AM, Scheen AJ, et al. Effects of the cannabinoid-1 receptor blocker rimonabant on weight reduction and cardiovascular risk factors in overweight patients: 1-year experience from the RIO-Europe study. Lancet 2005;365(9468):1389–97.

Diabetic Gastroparesis and Its Impact on Glycemia

Jessica Chang, BND, MBBS[a,b], Christopher K. Rayner, MBBS, PhD[a,b],
Karen L. Jones, PhD[a,b], Michael Horowitz, MBBS, PhD[a,b],*

KEYWORDS

• Gastric emptying • Diabetes • Incretin

During the past approximately 25 years, there has been a substantial redefinition of concepts relating to the prevalence, clinical significance, pathogenesis and management of disordered gastric motor function in diabetes. The application of novel diagnostic techniques has been fundamental to the achievement of these advances in knowledge. For example, diabetic gastroparesis was once considered a rare disorder associated with a poor prognosis,[1] but the use of radionuclide techniques has established that delayed gastric emptying occurs frequently in patients with long-standing type 1 or type 2 diabetes mellitus[2–5] and, at least in the majority of cases, does not seem to have a major effect on mortality.[6]

Diabetes is the most common cause of chronic gastroparesis. Furthermore, upper gastrointestinal symptoms occur frequently in diabetes and represent a hitherto underestimated cause of morbidity, as was the case with erectile dysfunction in male diabetics. Moreover, the number of hospitalizations occurring as a result of symptomatic gastroparesis is apparently increasing.[7] Hence, it is not surprising that the major focus of research studies has hitherto related to the etiology of gastrointestinal symptoms, in particular their relationship with delayed gastric emptying, and strategies for their therapeutic management.[8,9] It is only recently that there has been a shift in direction with the recognition that the rate of gastric emptying is a major determinant of both postprandial glycemia[10,11] and blood pressure.[12]

This article summarizes recent advances in knowledge relating to diabetic gastroparesis, with particular emphasis on the impact of normal and disordered gastric emptying on postprandial glycemic excursions and consequent dietary and pharmacologic strategies to improve chronic glycemic control by modulating gastric emptying.

[a] Discipline of Medicine, Level 6, Eleanor Harrald Building, Royal Adelaide Hospital, University of Adelaide, South Australia 5000, Australia
[b] Centre of Clinical Research Excellence in Nutritional Physiology, Interventions, and Outcomes, Adelaide, South Australia, Australia
* Corresponding author. Discipline of Medicine, Level 6, Eleanor Harrald Building, Royal Adelaide Hospital, University of Adelaide, South Australia 5000, Australia.
E-mail address: michael.horowitz@adelaide.edu.au

Endocrinol Metab Clin N Am 39 (2010) 745–762
doi:10.1016/j.ecl.2010.08.007
0889-8529/10/$ – see front matter © 2010 Elsevier Inc. All rights reserved.
endo.theclinics.com

PREVALENCE AND PROGNOSIS

The true prevalence of diabetic gastroparesis remains uncertain because of the absence of population-based studies and inconsistencies in definition.[1] There have been attempts to define gastroparesis, or gastropathy on the basis of the presence of upper gastrointestinal symptoms alone when other causes, including gastric outlet obstruction, have been excluded.[1,13,14] The authors believe this is inappropriate given that the relationship between symptoms and the rate of gastric emptying is, at best, weak[1] and abnormally delayed gastric emptying may be relevant even in the absence of gut symptoms (eg, as a cause of unstable glycemic control in insulin-treated patients). Many test meals have been used to measure gastric emptying in patients with diabetes with consequent substantial variation in the reported normal range.[9] When objectively determined, it seems that approximately 30% to 50% of long-standing patients with type 1 and 2 diabetes mellitus have gastroparesis, with a comparable prevalence in both type 1 and type 2 patients.[2–5,15] In many cases, the magnitude of the delay in gastric emptying is modest,[16] suggesting that it may be logical to stratify gastroparesis according to its severity. Gastric emptying is also not infrequently abnormally rapid, perhaps particularly in tertiary referral cases.[17]

The prognosis of diabetic gastroparesis has been assumed to be poor; however, few data in a small cohort followed for a mean period of 12 years suggest that this is not necessarily the case, with no major deterioration in either the rate of emptying or symptoms over this time period.[16]

PATHOPHYSIOLOGY

Normal gastric emptying is dependent on the integration of motor activity of the proximal and distal stomach, pylorus, and the upper small intestine, which is controlled by electrical slow waves generated by the so-called interstitial cells of Cajal, located in the myenteric plexus. The proximal stomach initially accommodates the meal, so that there is little increase in intragastric pressure. Subsequently, the antrum grinds and transports ingesta toward the pylorus where localized tonic and phasic pyloric contractile activity regulate flow. Emptying of nutrients from the stomach normally occurs at an overall rate of approximately 1 to 4 kcal per minute,[18] primarily as a result of inhibitory feedback arising from the interaction of nutrients with receptors in the small intestine[19] resulting in relaxation of the fundus, suppression of antral contractions, and stimulation of tonic and phasic pyloric activity.[9] These effects are dependent on the length (and probably the region) of small intestine exposed to nutrient and are mediated by gut hormones, including cholecystokinin,[20] glucagon-like peptide-1 (GLP-1),[21] peptide YY,[22] as well as neural pathways.[8]

Diabetic gastroparesis is associated with heterogeneous motor dysfunctions, involving the proximal stomach, antrum, pylorus, and duodenum, and incoordination of the motor activity between these different regions of the stomach.[8] Although irreversible autonomic (vagal) neuropathy has been widely regarded as the underlying cause of these motor abnormalities/gastroparesis, recent insights gained from examination of gastric tissue from a small number of patients with diabetic gastroparesis and animal models indicate a heterogeneous pathologic picture associated with abnormalities in multiple, interreacting cell types, including reduced numbers of interstitial cells of Cajal,[23,24] deficiencies of inhibitory neurotransmission,[23,24] decreased number of extrinsic autonomic neurons,[25] smooth muscle fibrosis,[23] and abnormalities in the function of immune cells. Loss and/or dysfunction of the interstitial cells of Cajal seems central to the pathogenesis of diabetic gastroparesis.[26] Data from the recently established National Institutes of Health–funded Gastroparesis Clinical Research

Consortium indicate that in approximately 50% of patients with severe diabetic gastroparesis there is a substantial reduction in the number of interstitial cells of Cajal. Loss of neuronal nitric oxide synthase expression within the myenteric neurons leading to a reduction in intraneuronal levels of nitric oxide, an important neurotransmitter for the maintenance of gastric motility, is observed in animals and humans with diabetes. It may reflect inhibition of neuronal nitric oxide synthase by advanced glycation products and is not explicable solely on the basis of neuronal loss.[27] A reduction in levels of heme oxygenase-1, the enzyme that gives rise to carbon monoxide, which protects the interstitial cells of Cajal from oxidative stress, is evident in nonobese diabetic (NOD) mice with delayed gastric emptying.[28] A series of elegant studies by Farrugia and colleagues[28–30] has demonstrated in the NOD mouse (a model of type 1 diabetes mellitus) that administration of hemin, which increases expression of heme oxygenase-1[28,30] and administration of carbon monoxide[29] result in reversal of the loss of interstitial cells of Cajal and normalization of delayed gastric emptying. Hemin, which is used in the treatment of acute intermittent porphyria in humans, has been shown to increase plasma levels of heme oxygenase-1, when given intravenously to healthy humans.[31]

It is now recognized that acute variations in the blood glucose concentration have a major impact on gastric emptying in both healthy and diabetic subjects[32]—marked hyperglycemia (blood glucose approximately 15 mmol/L) slows gastric emptying of solids and liquids substantially.[33] Even at physiologic postprandial glycemia (approximately 8 mmol/L), gastric emptying is slower when compared with euglycemia (blood glucose approximately 4 mmol/L) in both healthy subjects and patients with uncomplicated type 1 diabetes mellitus.[34] Acute hyperglycemia is associated with a reduction in fundal tone, suppression of antral contraction waves, increased pyloric contractions,[32] and induction of gastric electrical dysrhythmias.[35] Hyperglycemia may also increase the perception of gastrointestinal sensations (eg, the perception of fullness induced by gastric balloon distension is greater during hyperglycemia [blood glucose ≥15 mmol/L] when compared with euglycemia).[36] It should be recognized that no studies have evaluated the prevalence of diabetic gastroparesis during euglycemia. Hence, the reported prevalence is likely to represent an overestimate. As indicative of the substantial effect of hyperglycemia on gastric emptying and its clinical relevance, the acceleration of gastric emptying by prokinetic drugs used to treat gastroparesis (eg, erythromycin) is markedly impaired by hyperglycemia, even within the physiologic postprandial range.[37–39]

In contrast to the effects of hyperglycemia, gastric emptying is accelerated by insulin-induced hypoglycemia, even in type 1 diabetics with gastroparesis,[40] probably serving as a counter-regulatory mechanism to increase the delivery of nutrients for absorption.

DIAGNOSIS

In any patient with diabetes, upper gastrointestinal symptoms suggestive of delayed gastric emptying should be investigated to exclude reversible causes (**Box 1**). As discussed previously, the diagnosis of gastroparesis is usually based on the presence of upper gastrointestinal symptoms in combination with objective evidence of delayed gastric emptying[40]; the latter should ideally be measured during euglycemia, or at least with the blood glucose greater than 4 mmol/L and less than or equal to 10 mmol/L, given the effect of hyperglycemia to slow emptying.[33]

There are several techniques available to assess gastric emptying (summarized later). Of these methods, scintigraphy, which was established in the early 1980s, remains the gold standard.

Box 1
Causes of gastroparesis

Acute

    Drugs (eg, opiates, anticholinergics, levodopa, calcium channel blockers, β-blockers, octreotide, alcohol, nicotine, and cannabis)

    Electrolyte or metabolic disturbance (hyperglycemia, hypokalemia, and hypomagnesemia)

    Viral illness (gastroenteritis, *Herpes zoster* infection)

    Postoperative ileus

    Critical illness

Chronic

    Diabetes mellitus

    Idiopathic (including functional dyspepsia)

    Surgery (including vagotomy and heart and/or lung transplantation)

    Gastroesophageal reflux disease

    Achalasia

    Connective tissue diseases (systemic sclerosis, dermatomyositis or polymyositis, systemic lupus erythematosis, and amyloidosis)

    Endocrine or metabolic disturbance (hypothyroidism or hyperthyroidism, Addison disease, porphyria, and chronic liver or renal failure)

    Chronic idiopathic intestinal pseudo-obstruction

    Neuromuscular conditions (central nervous system disease, including stroke, trauma, or tumor; brainstem or spinal cord lesions; Parkinson disease; autonomic degeneration; and myotonic and muscular dystrophy)

    Anorexia nervosa

    Irradiation

    Neoplasia

    Infection (HIV and Chagas disease)

Data from Rayner CK, Horowitz M. New management approaches for gastroparesis. Nat Clin Pract Gastroenterol Hepatol 2005;2:454–62 [quiz: 93].

SCINTIGRAPHY

Using scintigraphy, the emptying time and intragastric distribution of solid and/or liquid meal components can be evaluated.[41] There have been increasing efforts to standardize the test meal and technique between centers. A recent consensus statement recommends the use of a low fat, egg white meal labeled with ^{99m}Tc-sulfur colloid consumed with jam and toast as a sandwich. and a glass of water. Gastric emptying is monitored for 4 hours after meal consumption; the intragastric retention at 4 hours has high sensitivity and specificity in diagnosis.[41] Despite this recommendation, scintigraphy is still not well standardized. Low-nutrient liquids should not be used to quantify gastric emptying for diagnostic purpose because they do not stimulate small intestinal feedback mechanisms, which are required to slow emptying.[42] Contrary to what is generally assumed, there is little, if any, evidence that the use of high-nutrient liquid or semisolid meals is inferior to solids. Moreover, the concurrent measurement of solid and nutrient liquid emptying may add diagnostic value, because in patients with diabetes the relationship between gastric emptying of solids and nutrient liquids is poor.[2]

STABLE ISOTOPE BREATH TEST

This noninvasive breath test has good reproducibility and the results have been reported to correlate well with scintigraphy, with a sensitivity and specificity of 86% and 80%, respectively, for the presence of delayed gastric emptying.[43] Breath tests use ^{13}C-acetate or ^{13}C-octanoate as a label and, in contrast to scintigraphy, do not involve exposure to ionising radiation. Furthermore, they are easy to administer and inexpensive.[44,45] After ingestion, the labeled meal passes through the stomach to the small intestine, where the ^{13}C-acetate or ^{13}C-octanoate is absorbed, metabolized into $^{13}CO_2$ in the liver, and exhaled via the breath. $^{13}CO_2$ in breath samples is analyzed by mass spectrometry.[44,45] Although this technique has advantages over scintigraphy, information relating to the validity of breath tests in patients with markedly delayed gastric emptying is limited.

OTHER DIAGNOSTIC METHODS

2-D ultrasonography is a valid, noninvasive, and convenient method to measure the emptying of liquids or semisolids, as well as antral contractions and transpyloric flow.[46,47] The more recently applied 3-D ultrasonography has the capacity to provide comprehensive imaging of the stomach, including information about intragastric meal distribution, and has been validated against scintigraphy to measure gastric emptying in both healthy subjects and patients with diabetic gastroparesis.[48] Although ultrasonography is readily available and does not involve exposure to radiation, obesity, abdominal gas, and the need for an experienced operator limit its widespread use.

MRI is another noninvasive way of measuring gastric emptying and motility; however, its use is limited to research purposes because of its high cost and limited availability.[49,50]

Swallowed capsule telemetry (Smart Pill) uses an ingestible capsule that measures intraluminal pH and pressure to determine the gastric emptying rate. This method has been reported to correlate well with scintigraphy with good sensitivity (82%) and specificity (83%)[51] but has not been used widely. Emptying of the capsule presumably occurs after that of digestible meal components.

The frequency of the gastric slow wave, which is normally approximately 3 cycles per minute, can be measured using surface electrodes attached to the skin of the epigastrium, so-called electrogastrography.[52] Although it is clear that abnormalities in gastric electrical activity, in particular tachygastria, occur frequently in diabetic gastroparesis[53] and may be induced by hyperglycemia,[35] the relationship is not sufficiently strong to be of diagnostic value.

Antropyloroduodenal manometry, using a water-perfused or solid-state catheter to measure intraluminal pressures in the stomach, pylorus, and small intestine, is only available in a few centers and remains primarily a research tool.

Paracetamol (acetaminophen) absorption test as a simple bedside test of gastric emptying is not advocated as a diagnostic tool because its use is limited to the gastric emptying of liquids and its accuracy is variable at best.[54]

SEQUELAE OF GASTROPARESIS

Gastroparesis, and possibly more rapid gastric emptying, in diabetes may be associated with upper gastrointestinal symptoms, such as nausea, vomiting, early satiety, postprandial fullness, bloating and abdominal pain[9] (the latter is often overlooked as a predominant symptom), and impaired regulation of postprandial glycemia and blood pressure.[5,12] The management of gastroparesis associated with upper gastrointestinal symptoms often involves a combination of dietary modification, prokinetic agents, and antiemetic drugs. In general, although the outcome of short-term, uncontrolled studies has been favorable, longer-term, controlled studies have frequently been negative; the withdrawal of cisapride (or marked restrictions in its availability) has left a major gap that has not, hitherto, been filled. Dietary recommendations have included increasing the liquid content of the meal, minimizing fat and fiber, vitamized diets, eating small and frequent meals, and avoiding alcohol, but none of these measures has been evaluated formally.[42,55] When an adequate oral intake cannot be achieved, nasojejunal feeding may prove successful, provided that small intestinal motility/secretory function is not severely disturbed, and this approach is preferable to parenteral nutrition.[13]

There is currently no evidence that recently developed antiemetics are any more effective than older drugs, such as prochlorperazine. Prokinetic agents, such as metoclopramide, erythromycin, and domperidone, may accelerate gastric emptying by increasing antral contractility and improving the organization of gastropyloroduodenal motility.[9] The relationship between their effects on symptoms and gastric emptying is, however, poor and there are few long-term studies. The use of metoclopramide subcutaneously is ideally suited to insulin-treated patients but the hazard of tardive dyskinesia, albeit rare, has led to increased concerns of its use (a box warning was issued by the Food and Drug Administration in 2009), so that domperidone may be regarded as the first-line drug in those countries in which it is available. Erythromycin, a macrolide antibiotic, mediates its effect on gastric emptying via its action as a motilin-receptor agonist, but its long-term use is limited by tachyphylaxis, gastrointestinal adverse effects, and increased risk of cardiac death with certain drug interactions, which has led to the recent development of motilin-receptor agonists without antimicrobial properties.[9] Glycemic control must be optimized in diabetics to minimize exacerbation of symptoms by hyperglycemia and potential attenuation of the effect of prokinetic drugs. This may require insulin pump therapy and, possibly, the use of low-carbohydrate diets.

Despite the initial promise of intrapyloric botulinum toxin,[56,57] randomized, controlled trials of this therapy have shown improvement in neither the rate of gastric emptying nor provision of symptom relief.[58,59]

Gastric electrical stimulation (GES) involves the implantation of electrodes in the smooth muscle layer of the gastric wall by laparotomy or laparoscopy, which are connected to a subcutaneously located pulse generator. Two types of stimulation have been evaluated in humans. One uses low-frequency, long-duration pulses, at or just above the frequency of gastric slow waves of 3 per minute pulses and the other uses high-frequency, short-duration pulses at four times the slow wave frequency (12 per minute).[13] The latter mode is used in the commercially available Enterra device but does not entrain the slow wave or markedly affect gastric emptying; rather, the rationale is that symptoms of nausea and vomiting might be improved by stimulation of afferent nerves. Benefits of GES have been reported in several uncontrolled case series[60-62] but in a recent double-blind trial with GES in diabetic gastroparesis, although there was an initial symptomatic improvement in the run-in "on" phase, the subsequent phase randomized to "on" or "off" showed no significant differences between the two.[63] Therefore, GES requires further evaluation in well-designed clinical trials before it can be recommended. Several different forms of GES are in development.

The benefits of surgical therapy for intractable gastroparesis, such as insertion of venting gastrostomy, partial or complete gastrectomy and reconstruction, or pancreatic transplantation, are uncertain because reported case series involve small numbers and have been uncontrolled. Surgery, usually involving partial gastrectomy, should only be performed in specialized centers with expertise in this area.[14,64,65]

There is a need for novel therapeutic approaches to gastroparesis because there is a lack of effective therapy for this common and debilitating disorder. The future holds promise with several drugs with different pharmacologic properties in development. These include the motilin agonist, mitemcinal,[66] ghrelin and ghrelin receptor agonists,[67,68] serotonin receptor agonists; and the muscarinic M1/M2 antagonist, acotiamide.[69]

POSTPRANDIAL HYPOTENSION

There is a significant relationship between the rate of gastric emptying and postprandial blood pressure—postprandial hypotension, defined as a fall in blood pressure greater than 20 mm Hg, occurring within 2 hours of a meal, occurs in approximately 40% of nursing home residents, especially in the elderly subgroup, and both type 1 and 2 diabetics with autonomic neuropathy (ie, a prevalence which is higher than that of orthostatic hypotension) and represents a major cause of morbidity (falls, angina, and stroke) and probably mortality.[70] More rapid gastric emptying results in a greater fall in blood pressure[12,70] so that in both the healthy elderly and patients with type 2 diabetes mellitus, the postprandial fall in blood pressure is attenuated when gastric emptying is slowed by dietary (eg, guar) or pharmacologic (eg, acarbose) means.[70,71] Conversely, gastric distension attenuates the fall in postprandial blood pressure.[70] Modulation of the rate of gastric emptying, therefore, has important therapeutic implications for the treatment of this condition on patients with diabetes which are yet to be explored adequately.

ROLE OF THE STOMACH IN GLUCOSE HOMEOSTASIS

It is not surprising that the stomach plays a pivotal role in normal blood glucose homeostasis given that it stores ingested nutrients and empties them into the small intestine at a tightly regulated rate, where they are digested and stimulate the release of the incretin hormones, glucose-dependent insulinotropic polypeptide (GIP) and GLP-1, which stimulate insulin secretion.[72] It is now recognized that the rate of gastric emptying (and probably small intestinal transit) is a major factor influencing postprandial glycemic excursions in health and in both type 1 and 2 diabetes.[72] Hence, gastric emptying is both a determinant of, as well as determined by, glycemia.[73]

Although it is well established that glycated hemoglobin is a measure of overall glycemic control and a marker of the development of microvascular and, to some extent, macrovascular complications of diabetes, the recognition that it is usually influenced more by postprandial than fasting glycemia, particularly when glycemic control is better, has occurred only recently.[74,75] This is despite the fact that the rationale for this is straightforward—because meals normally empty from the stomach at an overall rate of approximately 1 to 4 kcal per minute, only a small proportion of the day, perhaps 3 to 4 hours before breakfast, is truly reflective of the fasting glycemic state. In patients with diabetic gastroparesis, this period is likely even less.[9] Hence, the duration of postprandial glycemic excursions should not be equated with the duration of the postprandial state.

The incretin effect, which refers to the greater insulin response to an oral, when compared with an isoglycemic, glucose load, demonstrated in the early 1960s, is mediated by the gastrointestinal hormones, GLP-1, found predominantly in the distal small intestine and colon, and GIP, also known as gastric inhibitory polypeptide, which is secreted primarily from the proximal small intestine.[72] GLP-1 and GIP seem to be responsible for approximately 70% of the postprandial insulin response in healthy humans.[76] GLP-1 also lowers glucagon secretion and retards gastric emptying whereas GIP raises glucagon levels slightly and has no effect on gastric emptying.[77] In type 2 diabetes mellitus, the incretin effect is markedly reduced, probably representing an epiphenomenon[78] and this seems to be primarily because the capacity of GIP to augment insulin secretion is impaired, in part as a result of hyperglycemia[79–82] as the actions of GLP-1 are relatively preserved. It has been suggested that there may be a reduction in postprandial GLP-1 secretion, especially in those with long-standing diabetes,[78] but these latter studies have not taken into account the effect of variations in gastric emptying.

Plasma glucose concentrations begin to rise approximately 10 minutes after the start of a meal due to the absorption of dietary carbohydrates, and the peak glucose level in type 2 diabetics usually occurs at approximately 2 hours postprandially. The postprandial glucose profile is potentially influenced by several factors, including the preprandial glucose level, carbohydrate content of the meal, the rate of absorption, and insulin and glucagon secretion and their coordinated effects on glucose metabolism In the liver and peripheral tissues. Although the contribution of these factors to the postprandial glucose concentration is variable, the rate of gastric emptying has been shown to be a major determinant of the initial rise in blood glucose in both health[11] and in patients with type 1[83] and type 2 diabetes mellitus.[10] Initial studies demonstrated a relationship between the magnitude of the rise in blood glucose after oral glucose[11] and carbohydrate-containing meals[84] in health and type 2 diabetes mellitus.[84,85] When gastric emptying is more rapid, the rise in blood glucose is greater. In type 1 diabetics, a reduced amount of insulin is required to maintain euglycemia in the first 2 hours after a meal in patients with gastroparesis when compared with those with normal gastric emptying.[86]

It had been assumed that the relationship of glycemia with small intestinal carbohydrate delivery was linear, but this has recently been shown not to be the case.[87] When glucose is infused intraduodenally at rates within the normal range for gastric emptying in both healthy subjects[87] and type 2 patients,[88] there is only a modest rise in blood glucose when the infusion rate is 1 kcal per minute, a substantial rise in response to 2 kcal per minute, and little further increment when the rate is increased to 4 kcal per minute (**Fig. 1**). These discrepant responses are accounted for by the substantially increased plasma insulin response to the 4 kcal per minute infusion, which, in turn, is explicable on the basis of incretin hormone secretion.[87] There seems to be minimal contribution of GLP-1 toward the incretin effect at low caloric loads (ie, at 1 kcal/min there is minimal, transient, stimulation of GLP-1 compared with sustained elevation in GIP). In contrast, at higher rates of glucose delivery of 4 kcal per minute, although GIP increases further, there is a dramatic increase in GLP-1 secretion.[72,87] Accordingly, the former is likely to be responsible for the marked increase in insulin.[72] The implications are that GLP-1 is of particular importance at higher rates of duodenal glucose delivery and when the rate of gastric emptying is less than 1 kcal per minute in health and type 2 diabetes mellitus, there is little rise in blood glucose.

In both healthy and type 2 diabetic subjects, initially more rapid delivery of glucose to the small intestine results in higher GIP, GLP-1, and insulin responses when compared with a constant delivery of an identical glucose load. This early increase in insulin response, however, is unable to compensate for the greater initial rise in absorbed glucose, resulting in poor overall glycemic control, suggesting that this approach would not prove effective therapeutically.[89,90]

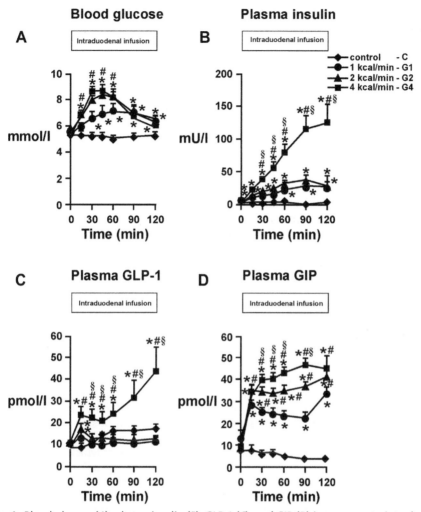

Fig. 1. Blood glucose (A), plasma insulin (B), GLP-1 (C), and GIP (D) in response to intraduodenal glucose (25%, 1390 mOsm/L) infused over 120 minutes at rates of 1 (G1), 2 (G2), or 4 (G4) kcal/min, or saline (4.2%, 1390 mOsm/L) control (C) in 10 healthy men. (A) *, Versus control: $P<.05$; #, versus G1: $P<.05$; §, versus G2: $P<.05$. (B) *, Versus control: $P<.05$; #, versus G1: $P<.05$; §, versus G2: $P<.05$. (C) *, Versus control: $P<.05$; #, versus G1: $P<.05$; §, versus G2: $P<.05$. (D) *, Versus control: $P<.05$; #, versus G1: $P<.05$; §, versus G2: $P<.05$. Data are means ± SEM. (Adapted from Pilichiewicz AN, Chaikomin R, Brennan IM, et al. Load-dependent effects of duodenal glucose on glycemia, gastrointestinal hormones, antropyloroduodenal motility, and energy intake in healthy men. Am J Physiol Endocrinol Metab 2007;293(3): E743–53; with permission.)

MODULATION OF GASTRIC EMPTYING TO IMPROVE GLYCEMIC CONTROL

The understanding that gastric emptying is an important determinant of postprandial glycemia has stimulated the development of dietary and pharmacologic approaches to improve overall glycemic control via modulating gastric emptying. The underlying strategies vary between diabetics who are treated with insulin and those who are not (type 2), with the focus on co-ordination of insulin administration and nutrient delivery in the former and retardation of gastric emptying in the latter, as long as it is not associated with the induction of upper gastrointestinal symptoms. In insulin-treated patients, gastroparesis may lead to otherwise unexplained hypoglycemia, particularly early in the postprandial period (so-called gastric hypoglycemia).[91,92] The outcome of recent studies using duodenal glucose infusion suggests that in non-insulin-treated patients it would be desirable for the rate of gastric emptying to be less than or equal to 1 kcal per minute for there to be minimal rise in postprandial glucose levels.[88,89]

DIETARY STRATEGIES

Dietary strategies designed to slow carbohydrate absorption include an increase in soluble fiber,[93] addition of the nonabsorbable polysaccharide—guar gum[94] and consumption of a nutrient preload before a carbohydrate meal.[95] The rationale underlying the latter approach is to slow gastric emptying of the meal by stimulating small intestinal hormonal and neural feedback mechanisms and stimulate the release of GLP-1.[95] It was initially shown that an olive oil preload delays gastric emptying and the postprandial rise in blood glucose but exerts only a modest effect on the peak blood glucose reponse.[95] In contrast, acute administration of a whey protein preload reduces the peak glucose level and overall glucose response substantially (**Fig. 2**), because, in addition to slowing gastric emptying and stimulating GIP and GLP-1, there is substantial stimulation of insulin secretion, probably mediated by amino acids.[96] Although the chronic effects of protein preloads on glycemia remain to be determined, the approach is promising.

Pharmacologic agents have also been developed with the aim of controlling postprandial glycemia by modulating gastric emptying. Pramlintide, an amylin analog, improves postprandial glycemia in both patients with type 1 and 2 diabetes mellitus by slowing gastric emptying[97,98] and also suppresses both postprandial glucagon secretion and appetite.[99]

Analogs of GLP-1 are now used widely in the management of type 2 diabetes mellitus and, although it is well documented that exogenous GLP-1 slows gastric emptying markedly,[100] the potential effects of these drugs on gastric emptying have received inappropriately little attention. It has been shown that retardation of gastric emptying makes a significant contribution to the effect of exenatide in reducing postprandial glycemia in patients with type 2 diabetes mellitus, at least acutely.[100,101] The suppression of appetite and weight loss induced by these agents is probably unrelated to their effect on gastric motility.[101,102] The actions of both pramlintide and exenatide to slow gastric emptying are thought to be mediated via the vagus nerve[97,103] and there is evidence that the slowing of gastric emptying and consequent reduction in postprandial glycemia induced by exenatide are related to the rate of gastric emptying (ie, the magnitude of the slowing and reduction in glycemic excursions are less marked when gastric emptying is slower).[101] Whether or not this observed reduction in gastric emptying is evident with prolonged use of exenatide warrants further investigation, specifically, the possibility of tachyphylaxis leading to a diminished effect in slowing of gastric emptying requires exclusion.

Dipeptidyl peptidase-4 inhibitors increase plasma concentrations of active GLP-1 and thus may be expected to slow gastric emptying, an effect that would be predicted to be influenced by meal composition and energy content, given that GLP-1 is a physiologic regulator of gastric emptying,[21] but the data to date are inconsistent and any effect on gastric emptying seems modest. This may reflect the effects of dipeptidyl

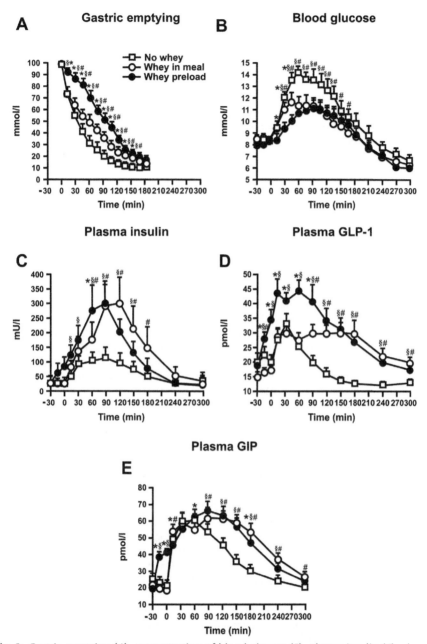

Fig. 2. Gastric emptying (*A*), concentration of blood glucose (*B*), plasma insulin (*C*), plasma GLP-1 (*D*), and plasma GIP (*E*) in response to a mashed potato meal in eight type 2 diabetic patients. In each study day, subjects ingested 350 mL of beef-flavored soup 30 minutes before a radiolabeled mashed potato meal; either 55 g of whey protein was added to the soup (whey preload) or no whey was given (no whey). Data are means ± SEM. *, *P*<.05: whey preload versus whey in meal; #, *P*<.05: whey in meal versus no whey; §, *P*<.05: whey preload versus no whey. (*Adapted from* Ma J, Stevens JE, Cukier K, et al. Effects of a protein preload on gastric emptying, glycemia, and gut hormones after a carbohydrate meal in diet-controlled type 2 diabetes. Diabetes Care 2009;32(9):1600–2; with permission.)

peptidase-4 inhibitors on other gut hormones, such as peptide YY or ghrelin, which neutralize the effect of GLP-1 elevation.[104]

SUMMARY

In recent years, there have been many advances in understanding the etiology of diabetic gastroparesis and the relevance of gastric emptying to glycemic control. The latter has translated to novel therapeutic strategies for the management of diabetes. The long-term efficacy of currently available therapeutic strategies and further developments in current experimental treatments, which use modulation of gastric emptying, are areas of ongoing research.

REFERENCES

1. Horowitz M, O'Donovan D, Jones KL, et al. Gastric emptying in diabetes: clinical significance and treatment. Diabet Med 2002;19(3):177–94.
2. Horowitz M, Maddox AF, Wishart JM, et al. Relationships between oesophageal transit and solid and liquid gastric emptying in diabetes mellitus. Eur J Nucl Med 1991;18(4):229–34.
3. Horowitz M, Wishart JM, Jones KL, et al. Gastric emptying in diabetes: an overview. Diabet Med 1996;13(9 Suppl 5):S16–22.
4. Horowitz M, Su YC, Rayner CK, et al. Gastroparesis: prevalence, clinical significance and treatment. Can J Gastroenterol 2001;15(12):805–13.
5. Jones KL, Horowitz M, Wishart MJ, et al. Relationships between gastric emptying, intragastric meal distribution and blood glucose concentrations in diabetes mellitus. J Nucl Med 1995;36(12):2220–8.
6. Kong MF, Horowitz M, Jones KL, et al. Natural history of diabetic gastroparesis. Diabetes Care 1999;22(3):503–7.
7. Wang YR, Fisher RS, Parkman HP. Gastroparesis-related hospitalizations in the United States: trends, characteristics, and outcomes, 1995–2004. Am J Gastroenterol 2008;103(2):313–22.
8. Ma J, Rayner CK, Jones KL, et al. Diabetic gastroparesis: diagnosis and management. Drugs 2009;69(8):971–86.
9. Khoo J, Rayner CK, Jones KL, et al. Pathophysiology and management of gastroparesis. Expert Rev Gastroenterol Hepatol 2009;3(2):167–81.
10. Jones KL, Horowitz M, Carney BI, et al. Gastric emptying in early noninsulin-dependent diabetes mellitus. J Nucl Med 1996;37(10):1643–8.
11. Horowitz M, Edelbroek MA, Wishart JM, et al. Relationship between oral glucose tolerance and gastric emptying in normal healthy subjects. Diabetologia 1993; 36(9):857–62.
12. Jones KL, Tonkin A, Horowitz M, et al. Rate of gastric emptying is a determinant of postprandial hypotension in non-insulin-dependent diabetes mellitus. Clin Sci (Lond) 1998;94(1):65–70.
13. Rayner CK, Horowitz M. New management approaches for gastroparesis. Nat Clin Pract Gastroenterol Hepatol 2005;2(10):454–62; [quiz: 93].
14. Jones MP, Maganti K. A systematic review of surgical therapy for gastroparesis. Am J Gastroenterol 2003;98(10):2122–9.
15. Samsom M, Vermeijden JR, Smout AJ, et al. Prevalence of delayed gastric emptying in diabetic patients and relationship to dyspeptic symptoms: a prospective study in unselected diabetic patients. Diabetes Care 2003; 26(11):3116–22.

16. Jones KL, Russo A, Berry MK, et al. A longitudinal study of gastric emptying and upper gastrointestinal symptoms in patients with diabetes mellitus. Am J Med 2002;113(6):449–55.

17. Bharucha AE, Camilleri M, Forstrom LA, et al. Relationship between clinical features and gastric emptying disturbances in diabetes mellitus. Clin Endocrinol (Oxf) 2009;70(3):415–20.

18. Brener W, Hendrix TR, McHugh PR. Regulation of the gastric emptying of glucose. Gastroenterology 1983;85(1):76–82.

19. Lin HC, Doty JE, Reedy TJ, et al. Inhibition of gastric emptying by glucose depends on length of intestine exposed to nutrient. Am J Physiol 1989; 256(2 Pt 1):G404–11.

20. Fried M, Erlacher U, Schwizer W, et al. Role of cholecystokinin in the regulation of gastric emptying and pancreatic enzyme secretion in humans. Studies with the cholecystokinin-receptor antagonist loxiglumide. Gastroenterology 1991; 101(2):503–11.

21. Deane AM, Nguyen NQ, Stevens JE, et al. Endogenous glucagon-like peptide-1 slows gastric emptying in healthy subjects, attenuating postprandial glycemia. J Clin Endocrinol Metab 2010;95(1):215–21.

22. Horowitz M, Jones KL, Akkermans LM, et al. Gastric function. In: Horowitz MSM, editor. Gastrointestinal function in diabetes mellitus. Chichester (United Kingdom): John Wiley & Sons Ltd; 2004. p. 117–76.

23. Pasricha PJ, Pehlivanov ND, Gomez G, et al. Changes in the gastric enteric nervous system and muscle: a case report on two patients with diabetic gastroparesis. BMC Gastroenterol 2008;8:21.

24. He CL, Soffer EE, Ferris CD, et al. Loss of interstitial cells of Cajal and inhibitory innervation in insulin-dependent diabetes. Gastroenterology 2001;121(2): 427–34.

25. Samsom M, Akkermans LM, Jebbink RJ, et al. Gastrointestinal motor mechanisms in hyperglycaemia induced delayed gastric emptying in type I diabetes mellitus. Gut 1997;40(5):641–6.

26. Forster J, Damjanov I, Lin Z, et al. Absence of the interstitial cells of Cajal in patients with gastroparesis and correlation with clinical findings. J Gastrointest Surg 2005;9(1):102–8.

27. Watkins CC, Sawa A, Jaffrey S, et al. Insulin restores neuronal nitric oxide synthase expression and function that is lost in diabetic gastropathy. J Clin Invest 2000;106(3):373–84.

28. Choi KM, Gibbons SJ, Nguyen TV, et al. Heme oxygenase-1 protects interstitial cells of Cajal from oxidative stress and reverses diabetic gastroparesis. Gastroenterology 2008;135(6):2055–64, 64 e1–2.

29. Kashyap PC, Choi KM, Dutta N, et al. Carbon monoxide reverses diabetic gastroparesis in NOD mice. Am J Physiol Gastrointest Liver Physiol 2010;298(6): G1013–9.

30. Choi KM, Kashyap PC, Dutta N, et al. CD206-positive M2 macrophages that express heme oxygenase-1 protect against diabetic gastroparesis in mice. Gastroenterology 2010;138(7):2399–409.

31. Bharucha AE, Kulkarni A, Choi KM, et al. First-in-human study demonstrating pharmacological activation of heme oxygenase-1 in humans. Clin Pharmacol Ther 2010;87(2):187–90.

32. Rayner CK, Samsom M, Jones KL, et al. Relationships of upper gastrointestinal motor and sensory function with glycemic control. Diabetes Care 2001;24(2): 371–81.

33. Fraser RJ, Horowitz M, Maddox AF, et al. Hyperglycaemia slows gastric emptying in type 1 (insulin-dependent) diabetes mellitus. Diabetologia 1990; 33(11):675–80.

34. Schvarcz E, Palmer M, Aman J, et al. Physiological hyperglycemia slows gastric emptying in normal subjects and patients with insulin-dependent diabetes mellitus. Gastroenterology 1997;113(1):60–6.

35. Jebbink RJ, Samsom M, Bruijs PP, et al. Hyperglycemia induces abnormalities of gastric myoelectrical activity in patients with type I diabetes mellitus. Gastroenterology 1994;107(5):1390–7.

36. Hebbard GS, Samsom M, Sun WM, et al. Hyperglycemia affects proximal gastric motor and sensory function during small intestinal triglyceride infusion. Am J Physiol 1996;271(5 Pt 1):G814–9.

37. Rayner CK, Su YC, Doran SM, et al. The stimulation of antral motility by erythromycin is attenuated by hyperglycemia. Am J Gastroenterol 2000; 95(9):2233–41.

38. Jones KL, Berry M, Kong MF, et al. Hyperglycemia attenuates the gastrokinetic effect of erythromycin and affects the perception of postprandial hunger in normal subjects. Diabetes Care 1999;22(2):339–44.

39. Jones KL, Kong MF, Berry MK, et al. The effect of erythromycin on gastric emptying is modified by physiological changes in the blood glucose concentration. Am J Gastroenterol 1999;94(8):2074–9.

40. Russo A, Stevens JE, Chen R, et al. Insulin-induced hypoglycemia accelerates gastric emptying of solids and liquids in long-standing type 1 diabetes. J Clin Endocrinol Metab 2005;90(8):4489–95.

41. Abell TL, Camilleri M, Donohoe K, et al. Consensus recommendations for gastric emptying scintigraphy: a joint report of the American Neurogastroenterology and Motility Society and the Society of Nuclear Medicine. J Nucl Med Technol 2008;36(1):44–54.

42. Wright RA, Clemente R, Wathen R. Diabetic gastroparesis: an abnormality of gastric emptying of solids. Am J Med Sci 1985;289(6):240–2.

43. Viramontes BE, Kim DY, Camilleri M, et al. Validation of a stable isotope gastric emptying test for normal, accelerated or delayed gastric emptying. Neurogastroenterol Motil 2001;13(6):567–74.

44. Chew CG, Bartholomeusz FD, Bellon M, et al. Simultaneous 13C/14C dual isotope breath test measurement of gastric emptying of solid and liquid in normal subjects and patients: comparison with scintigraphy. Nucl Med Rev Cent East Eur 2003;6(1):29–33.

45. Sanaka M, Urita Y, Sugimoto M, et al. Comparison between gastric scintigraphy and the [^{13}C]-acetate breath test with Wagner-Nelson analysis in humans. Clin Exp Pharmacol Physiol 2006;33(12):1239–43.

46. Hveem K, Jones KL, Chatterton BE, et al. Scintigraphic measurement of gastric emptying and ultrasonographic assessment of antral area: relation to appetite. Gut 1996;38(6):816–21.

47. Gilja OH, Hausken T, degaard S, et al. Gastric emptying measured by ultrasonography. World J Gastroenterol 1999;5(2):93–4.

48. Gentilcore D, Hausken T, Horowitz M, et al. Measurements of gastric emptying of low- and high-nutrient liquids using 3D ultrasonography and scintigraphy in healthy subjects. Neurogastroenterol Motil 2006;18(12):1062–8.

49. Kunz P, Feinle C, Schwizer W, et al. Assessment of gastric motor function during the emptying of solid and liquid meals in humans by MRI. J Magn Reson Imaging 1999;9(1):75–80.

50. Schwizer W, Fraser R, Borovicka J, et al. Measurement of gastric emptying and gastric motility by magnetic resonance imaging (MRI). Dig Dis Sci 1994; 39(Suppl 12):101S–3S.
51. Kuo B, McCallum RW, Koch KL, et al. Comparison of gastric emptying of a non-digestible capsule to a radio-labelled meal in healthy and gastroparetic subjects. Aliment Pharmacol Ther 2008;27(2):186–96.
52. Verhagen MA, Van Schelven LJ, Samsom M, et al. Pitfalls in the analysis of electrogastrographic recordings. Gastroenterology 1999;117(2):453–60.
53. Parkman HP, Hasler WL, Barnett JL, et al. Electrogastrography: a document prepared by the gastric section of the American Motility Society Clinical GI Motility Testing Task Force. Neurogastroenterol Motil 2003;15(2):89–102.
54. Willems M, Quartero AO, Numans ME. How useful is paracetamol absorption as a marker of gastric emptying? A systematic literature study. Dig Dis Sci 2001; 46(10):2256–62.
55. Olausson EA, Alpsten M, Larsson A, et al. Small particle size of a solid meal increases gastric emptying and late postprandial glycaemic response in diabetic subjects with gastroparesis. Diabetes Res Clin Pract 2008;80(2):231–7.
56. Lacy BE, Zayat EN, Crowell MD, et al. Botulinum toxin for the treatment of gastroparesis: a preliminary report. Am J Gastroenterol 2002;97(6):1548–52.
57. Miller LS, Szych GA, Kantor SB, et al. Treatment of idiopathic gastroparesis with injection of botulinum toxin into the pyloric sphincter muscle. Am J Gastroenterol 2002;97(7):1653–60.
58. Arts J, Holvoet L, Caenepeel P, et al. Clinical trial: a randomized-controlled crossover study of intrapyloric injection of botulinum toxin in gastroparesis. Aliment Pharmacol Ther 2007;26(9):1251–8.
59. Friedenberg FK, Palit A, Parkman HP, et al. Botulinum toxin A for the treatment of delayed gastric emptying. Am J Gastroenterol 2008;103(2):416–23.
60. McCallum RW, Chen JD, Lin Z, et al. Gastric pacing improves emptying and symptoms in patients with gastroparesis. Gastroenterology 1998;114(3): 456–61.
61. Abell T, McCallum R, Hocking M, et al. Gastric electrical stimulation for medically refractory gastroparesis. Gastroenterology 2003;125(2):421–8.
62. O'Grady G, Egbuji JU, Du P, et al. High-frequency gastric electrical stimulation for the treatment of gastroparesis: a meta-analysis. World J Surg 2009;33(8): 1693–701.
63. McCallum R, Brody F, Parkman HP, et al. Enterra gastric electrical stimulation for diabetic gastroparesis:results from a multicenter randomized study. Gastroenterology 2009;136:A61–2.
64. Ejskjaer NT, Bradley JL, Buxton-Thomas MS, et al. Novel surgical treatment and gastric pathology in diabetic gastroparesis. Diabet Med 1999;16(6): 488–95.
65. Watkins PJ, Buxton-Thomas MS, Howard ER. Long-term outcome after gastrectomy for intractable diabetic gastroparesis. Diabet Med 2003;20(1):58–63.
66. Takanashi H, Cynshi O. Motilides: a long and winding road: lessons from mitemcinal (GM-611) on diabetic gastroparesis. Regul Pept 2009;155(1–3):18–23.
67. Ejskjaer N, Vestergaard ET, Hellstrom PM, et al. Ghrelin receptor agonist (TZP-101) accelerates gastric emptying in adults with diabetes and symptomatic gastroparesis. Aliment Pharmacol Ther 2009;29(11):1179–87.
68. Murray CD, Martin NM, Patterson M, et al. Ghrelin enhances gastric emptying in diabetic gastroparesis: a double blind, placebo controlled, crossover study. Gut 2005;54(12):1693–8.

69. Parkman HP, Camilleri M, Farrugia G, et al. Gastroparesis and functional dyspepsia: excerpts from the AGA/ANMS meeting. Neurogastroenterol Motil 2010;22(2):113–33.
70. Gentilcore D, Jones KL, O'Donovan DG, et al. Postprandial hypotension – novel insights into pathophysiology and therapeutic implications. Curr Vasc Pharmacol 2006;4(2):161–71.
71. Gentilcore D, Bryant B, Wishart JM, et al. Acarbose attenuates the hypotensive response to sucrose and slows gastric emptying in the elderly. Am J Med 2005; 118(11):1289.
72. Ma J, Rayner CK, Jones KL, et al. Insulin secretion in healthy subjects and patients with type 2 diabetes—role of the gastrointestinal tract. Best Pract Res Clin Endocrinol Metab 2009;23(4):413–24.
73. Rayner CK, Horowitz M. Gastrointestinal motility and glycemic control in diabetes: the chicken and the egg revisited? J Clin Invest 2006;116(2):299–302.
74. Ceriello A, Hanefeld M, Leiter L, et al. Postprandial glucose regulation and diabetic complications. Arch Intern Med 2004;164(19):2090–5.
75. Monnier L, Lapinski H, Colette C. Contributions of fasting and postprandial plasma glucose increments to the overall diurnal hyperglycemia of type 2 diabetic patients: variations with increasing levels of HbA(1c). Diabetes Care 2003;26(3):881–5.
76. Horowitz M, Nauck MA. To be or not to be–an incretin or enterogastrone? Gut 2006;55(2):148–50.
77. Meier JJ. The contribution of incretin hormones to the pathogenesis of type 2 diabetes. Best Pract Res Clin Endocrinol Metab 2009;23(4):433–41.
78. Meier JJ, Nauck MA. Is the diminished incretin effect in type 2 diabetes just an epi-phenomenon of impaired beta-cell function? Diabetes 2010;59(5):1117–25.
79. Nauck MA, Heimesaat MM, Orskov C, et al. Preserved incretin activity of glucagon-like peptide 1 [7–36 amide] but not of synthetic human gastric inhibitory polypeptide in patients with type-2 diabetes mellitus. J Clin Invest 1993; 91(1):301–7.
80. Meier JJ, Hucking K, Holst JJ, et al. Reduced insulinotropic effect of gastric inhibitory polypeptide in first-degree relatives of patients with type 2 diabetes. Diabetes 2001;50(11):2497–504.
81. Meier JJ, Gallwitz B, Kask B, et al. Stimulation of insulin secretion by intravenous bolus injection and continuous infusion of gastric inhibitory polypeptide in patients with type 2 diabetes and healthy control subjects. Diabetes 2004; 53(Suppl 3):S220–4.
82. Vilsboll T, Krarup T, Madsbad S, et al. Defective amplification of the late phase insulin response to glucose by GIP in obese type II diabetic patients. Diabetologia 2002;45(8):1111–9.
83. Horowitz M, Harding PE, Maddox AF, et al. Gastric and oesophageal emptying in insulin-dependent diabetes mellitus. J Gastroenterol Hepatol 1986;1:97–113.
84. Wolever TM, Bolognesi C. Source and amount of carbohydrate affect postprandial glucose and insulin in normal subjects. J Nutr 1996;126(11):2798–806.
85. Pearce KL, Noakes M, Keogh J, et al. Effect of carbohydrate distribution on postprandial glucose peaks with the use of continuous glucose monitoring in type 2 diabetes. Am J Clin Nutr 2008;87(3):638–44.
86. Ishii M, Nakamura T, Kasai F, et al. Altered postprandial insulin requirement in IDDM patients with gastroparesis. Diabetes Care 1994;17(8):901–3.
87. Pilichiewicz AN, Chaikomin R, Brennan IM, et al. Load-dependent effects of duodenal glucose on glycemia, gastrointestinal hormones, antropyloroduodenal

motility, and energy intake in healthy men. Am J Physiol Endocrinol Metab 2007; 293(3):E743–53.

88. Rayner CK, Chapman MJ, Pilichiewicz A, et al. Effects of variations in duodenal glucose load on glycaemia, insulin and GLP-1 in type 2 diabetes (Abstract). Diabetologia 2009;52(Suppl 1):S105.

89. O'Donovan DG, Doran S, Feinle-Bisset C, et al. Effect of variations in small intestinal glucose delivery on plasma glucose, insulin, and incretin hormones in healthy subjects and type 2 diabetes. J Clin Endocrinol Metab 2004;89(7): 3431–5.

90. Chaikomin R, Doran S, Jones KL, et al. Initially more rapid small intestinal glucose delivery increases plasma insulin, GIP, and GLP-1 but does not improve overall glycemia in healthy subjects. Am J Physiol Endocrinol Metab 2005; 289(3):E504–7.

91. Lysy J, Israeli E, Strauss-Liviatan N, et al. Relationships between hypoglycaemia and gastric emptying abnormalities in insulin-treated diabetic patients. Neurogastroenterol Motil 2006;18(6):433–40.

92. Horowitz M, Jones KL, Rayner CK, et al. 'Gastric' hypoglycaemia—an important concept in diabetes management. Neurogastroenterol Motil 2006;18(6):405–7.

93. Chandalia M, Garg A, Lutjohann D, et al. Beneficial effects of high dietary fiber intake in patients with type 2 diabetes mellitus. N Engl J Med 2000;342(19): 1392–8.

94. Russo A, Stevens JE, Wilson T, et al. Guar attenuates fall in postprandial blood pressure and slows gastric emptying of oral glucose in type 2 diabetes. Dig Dis Sci 2003;48(7):1221–9.

95. Gentilcore D, Chaikomin R, Jones KL, et al. Effects of fat on gastric emptying of and the glycemic, insulin, and incretin responses to a carbohydrate meal in type 2 diabetes. J Clin Endocrinol Metab 2006;91(6):2062–7.

96. Ma J, Stevens JE, Cukier K, et al. Effects of a protein preload on gastric emptying, glycemia, and gut hormones after a carbohydrate meal in diet-controlled type 2 diabetes. Diabetes Care 2009;32(9):1600–2.

97. Vella A, Lee JS, Camilleri M, et al. Effects of pramlintide, an amylin analogue, on gastric emptying in type 1 and 2 diabetes mellitus. Neurogastroenterol Motil 2002;14(2):123–31.

98. Thompson RG, Pearson L, Schoenfeld SL, et al. Pramlintide, a synthetic analog of human amylin, improves the metabolic profile of patients with type 2 diabetes using insulin. The Pramlintide in Type 2 Diabetes Group. Diabetes Care 1998; 21(6):987–93.

99. Aronne L, Fujioka K, Aroda V, et al. Progressive reduction in body weight after treatment with the amylin analog pramlintide in obese subjects: a phase 2, randomized, placebo-controlled, dose-escalation study. J Clin Endocrinol Metab 2007;92(8):2977–83.

100. Little TJ, Pilichiewicz AN, Russo A, et al. Effects of intravenous glucagon-like peptide-1 on gastric emptying and intragastric distribution in healthy subjects: relationships with postprandial glycemic and insulinemic responses. J Clin Endocrinol Metab 2006;91(5):1916–23.

101. Linnebjerg H, Park S, Kothare PA, et al. Effect of exenatide on gastric emptying and relationship to postprandial glycemia in type 2 diabetes. Regul Pept 2008; 151(1–3):123–9.

102. Gutzwiller JP, Drewe J, Goke B, et al. Glucagon-like peptide-1 promotes satiety and reduces food intake in patients with diabetes mellitus type 2. Am J Physiol 1999;276(5 Pt 2):R1541–4.

103. Delgado-Aros S, Vella A, Camilleri M, et al. Effects of glucagon-like peptide-1 and feeding on gastric volumes in diabetes mellitus with cardio-vagal dysfunction. Neurogastroenterol Motil 2003;15(4):435–43.

104. Vella A, Bock G, Giesler PD, et al. The effect of dipeptidyl peptidase-4 inhibition on gastric volume, satiation and enteroendocrine secretion in type 2 diabetes: a double-blind, placebo-controlled crossover study. Clin Endocrinol (Oxf) 2008;69(5):737–44.

Harnessing the Pancreatic Stem Cell

David A. Taylor-Fishwick, PhD[a,b,*], Gary L. Pittenger, PhD[c,d]

KEYWORDS

- Pancreatic stem cell • Beta-cell mass • Differentiation
- Embryonic stem cells

Within the last decade, the collective view of the regenerative capacity of many organs has altered dramatically. The notion of being "born with your lot" is outdated because regenerative medicine represents one of the most aggressively expanding fields of translational research. The pancreas has offered a prime focus for these new endeavors because of the specialized cell types it contains and the significant health and economic consequences associated with the loss of the insulin-producing pancreatic beta cell. Widespread acceptance exists that clinical diabetes is associated with a loss of functional beta-cell mass. Although this loss of beta-cell mass is the dogma for type 1 diabetes, which is a consequence of an autoimmune Th1-mediated destruction of insulin-producing cells, recent studies have revealed that it is also a key factor in the development of type 2 diabetes. Islet loss is protracted in type 2 diabetes, occurring over a period of 10 to 15 years before diagnosis, during which there is a progressive infiltration of amyloid. Loss of islet mass occurs at a rate of 5% to 10% per year, which is a decline that continues even with postdiagnosis therapy.

Replacement of functional beta-cell mass is a logical approach to reverse diabetes. As illustrated in **Fig. 1**, several approaches are being championed to replace functional beta-cell mass. Transplantation, which is the most direct approach, has been extensively studied. Clinical trials of donor islet transplantation have effectively served the purpose of providing proof-of-concept data to show that restoring functional beta-cell mass reverses diabetes.[1] However, despite advances in immunosuppression

[a] Department of Internal Medicine, Strelitz Diabetes Center, LH 2128, 700 West Olney Road, Norfolk, VA 23507, USA
[b] Department of Microbiology and Molecular Cell Biology, LH 2128, 700 West Olney Road, Norfolk, VA 23507, USA
[c] Department of Internal Medicine, Strelitz Diabetes Center, 855 West Brambleton Avenue, Norfolk, VA 23510, USA
[d] Department of Anatomy and Pathology, Strelitz Diabetes Center, 855 West Brambleton Avenue, Norfolk, VA 23510, USA
* Corresponding author. Department of Internal Medicine, Strelitz Diabetes Center, LH 2128, 700 W Olney Road, Norfolk, VA 23507.
E-mail address: Taylord@evms.edu

Endocrinol Metab Clin N Am 39 (2010) 763–776
doi:10.1016/j.ecl.2010.08.008
0889-8529/10/$ – see front matter © 2010 Elsevier Inc. All rights reserved.

endo.theclinics.com

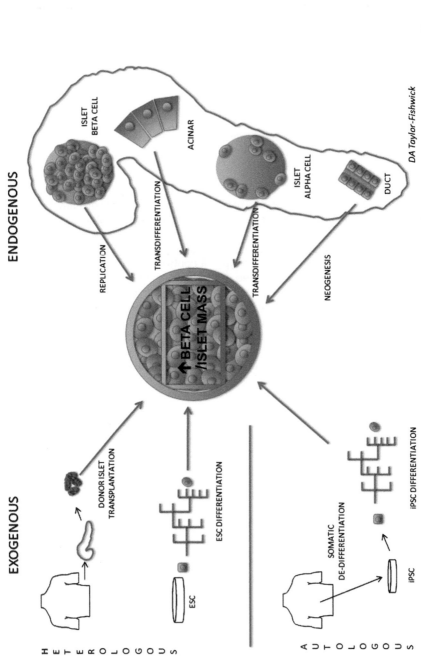

Fig. 1. Overview of the approaches to replace functional beta-cell mass. These include exogenous strategies (*left*), using heterologous (donor) material (*upper left*) from direct islet transplantation or embryonic stem cell (ESC) differentiation or autologous cells (*lower left*) reprogrammed as induced pluripotent stem cells (iPSCs) and redifferentiated. To the right, endogenous (self-pancreas derived) strategies are shown. These pathways and associated consideration are discussed in this article.

regimens,[1-5] prevascularized implantation sites,[6] and encapsulated barriers to protect islets,[7] long-term islet graft survival is limited. In addition, availability of donor islets is severely limited (donors available represent <0.1% of the need), and transplantation involves long-term exposure to toxic immunosuppressants.[8] Fueled by the conceptual success of diabetes reversal by increasing beta-cell mass through transplantation, alternative strategies to restore functional beta-cell mass are being aggressively studied.

Building on the elaborate research studies that have helped map out key decision points in the process of pancreas development, reprogramming of pluripotent embryonic stem cells (ESCs) or induced pluripotent stem cells (iPSCs) offers the possibility of overcoming restrictions on tissue supply associated with the transplantation of donor islets. In a healthy pancreas, the beta-cell mass can exhibit significant plasticity, as reflected in the normal adaptive response in beta-cell mass to offset the metabolic challenge associated with pregnancy and obesity.[9] Capitalizing on the innate plasticity of the pancreas, targeting precursor cells in the pancreas (adult stem cells) opens the opportunity to reprogram the pancreas in situ using pharmacologic intervention.

In this article, alternative strategies and potential sources of pancreatic stem cells are considered. The ability to exert control over functional beta-cell mass within the pancreas represents a "holy grail" in reversing diabetes. Harnessing the pancreatic stem cell is a likely option to realize several defined criteria of an ideal approach to repopulate pancreatic islets:

- Islets can be regenerated from endogenous cells.
- Islets should express a full complement of islet hormones, including counterregulatory hormones, such as glucagon, to prevent hypoglycemia.
- There is no need for immunotherapy or use of benign drugs.
- The treatment should be applicable to both type 1 and type 2 diabetes.
- Sufficient insulin production is required to combat the diabetes and insulin resistance.
- Insulin secretion should be regulated.
- The effect of treatment should persist beyond the treatment period
- The treatment should not be associated with toxicity.

PANCREAS CELL DIFFERENTIATION DURING DEVELOPMENT

The pancreas is an organ of heterogeneous cell types and functions.[10] Deriving from common pancreatic precursor progenitor cells located within the early gut endoderm, the adult pancreas consists of 3 main cell types, the exocrine acinar cells, endocrine cells, and epithelial cells of the ducts or ductules. After gastrulation, in the gut endoderm, 2 key transcription factors (Sonic and Indian Hedgehog) are expressed.[11,12] Repression of these hedgehog proteins is mediated by the contact of the foregut endoderm with the notochord. This interaction helps define the region destined to become the ventral pancreatic bud.[13,14] Activin B and fibroblast growth factor 2 are key mediators arising from the notochord, which repress the expression of hedgehog proteins.[12,15] Pancreatic precursor cells deriving from this endoderm specialization are defined by the expression of a variety of transcription factors, including Sox9, Ptf1a, Hlxb9, Pdx-1, and attainment of notch signaling.[16] Via an iterative process of lateral specification, notch-delta signaling provides a key step in determining pancreatic precursor cell fate.[17] Receipt of notch signaling is consistent with the expression of the bHLH transcription factor Hes1. Conversely, the cell sending the signal attains expression of the bHLH transcription factor neurogenin 3 (ngn3). Endocrine fate determination depends on the expression of ngn3,[18,19] as evidenced by the absence of all pancreatic endocrine cells in ngn3-null mice[18] and forced misexpression of ngn3, resulting in aberrant endocrine differentiation.[20] Reciprocally, expression of Hes-1 in the cell defines a nonendocrine cell fate.

Insulin expression is detected at 2 distinct phases in the developing pancreas anlagen. An initial first wave of endocrine cells, although expressing insulin, do not express the markers of mature endocrine cells.[21–24] A subsequent stage known as secondary transition is associated with a dramatic increase in endocrine cells budding from the pancreatic ductal epithelium (termed neogenesis). These endocrine cells differentiate from an ngn3-expressing precursor cell and contribute to the mature functional islet.

The ngn3-expressing cell is the precursor of the 5 identified endocrine cells in the islet,[18] the glucagon-producing alpha cell, insulin-producing beta cell, somatostatin-producing delta cell, pancreatic polypeptide–producing cell, and ghrelin-producing epsilon cell. Through an elegant series of gene deletion studies in mice, several key events required for the maturation of the ngn3 precursor to terminally differentiated endocrine cells have been identified.[13,14,25] Key transcription factors in the formation of beta and alpha cells include Pax4 and Arx.[26–28] These factors have opposing actions, and reciprocal binding sites for each other's promoter have been identified. Pax4, a paired homeodomain factor, is required during secondary transition for beta-cell differentiation. Pax4 is thought to function as a transcriptional repressor, binding the promoters and repressing the expression of ghrelin, glucagon, and Arx.[28–30] In contrast, Arx, which is downstream of ngn3, promotes alpha-cell development as evidenced in Arx-null mice that had a complete loss of alpha cells and a concomitant increase in beta cells.[28] Progression of beta-cell differentiation depends on the homeodomain factor Nkx2.2[31] because embryos with mutation in Nkx2.2 have no beta cells but retain alpha cells. The mature beta cell is characterized by an elevated expression of Pdx1, which is a transcription factor that is essential for beta-cell survival[32,33] and function[34–36] and binds and transactivates several genes including insulin.[37]

Although many of these pathways have been identified by gene deletion studies providing an informative all-or-nothing view, recent data using conditional knockdown experiments[38,39] identify gradients and thresholds of transcriptional expression as dictators of cell fate in endocrine differentiation. This added layer of sophistication underlies the challenge in approaches to recapitulate, in vitro, the conditions that occur during development to reprogram a pluripotent cell into a functional insulin-producing beta cell and/or islet.

REPROGRAMMING THE ESC

Differentiation of ESCs into insulin-producing cells offers great attraction as an alternative islet source. ESCs are undifferentiated cells with an unlimited self-renewal capacity and high plasticity.[40] Under the appropriate conditions, ESCs are responsive to extracellular signals and capable of differentiating into any cell type. Although this technique has huge potential, the challenge, as outlined earlier, is to identify and unlock the differentiation and islet commitment signals, determine their temporal sequence, and define the concentration that they need to be presented. Two global approaches have been championed to turn ESCs into insulin-producing cells, (1) to circumvent the myriad of differentiation signals and directly reprogram the ESC and (2) to coax ESCs through normal development checkpoints by recreating key differentiation steps.

In early studies, insulin-positive cells were identified in unstructured ESC differentiation (such as which occurs in embryoid body formation from ESCs). These insulin-positive cells appear to be immature, reminiscent of the insulin-expressing cell in the first phase of pancreatogenesis, and distinct from organized functional islets.[41–43] Moreover, the numbers of insulin-positive cells detected was low, approximately 1%. To enrich these spontaneously derived insulin-positive cells, a 5-step protocol was devised after the selection of embryoid body cells that expressed the intermediate filament nestin.[44] With further protocol modifications, the transplanted cells were able to restore euglycemia in diabetic mice.[45] However, the nature of these insulin-positive cells has been questioned after the realization that a significant proportion of the intracellular insulin may be derived by uptake from culture media rather than de novo synthesis.[46,47] Direct reprogramming of undifferentiated ESCs by the forced expression of key transcription regulators, such as Pdx1, ngn3, or Pax4,[48–51] has been championed, but given the developing data on the complex regulation in the derivation of endocrine cells in the normal pancreas, it is unclear if these strategies will promote stable changes and functional cells.

Logic suggests that the optimal path to achieving functional beta cells in large numbers would be to guide ESCs through the differentiation checkpoints that occur in utero. Development of a defined protocol with consistent outcomes is a prime milestone, limiting commercialization of this technology. A significant advance in achieving islets from ESCs has been the development of multistep differentiation processes that apply the discoveries in developmental biology to recapitulate beta-cell development[52]; especially key has been the identification of signals to derive definitive endoderm from ESCs. The generation of definitive endoderm, as defined by the expression of CXCR4 and Sox 17, has been achieved with combinations of activin and BMP4[53] or activin and sodium butyrate[54] or activin and Wnt.[42,55–57] Subsequent stimulation of definitive endoderm with cocktails of growth factors temporally spaced to promote key commitment steps in cell differentiation[52] has resulted in the generation of insulin-producing, glucose-sensitive cell clusters.[42,53,54,56] These islet-like clusters have been reported to produce insufficient insulin to reverse hyperglycemia in experimental models of diabetes and express markers that are consistent with first-wave insulin cells rather than insulin cells arising from the second transition.[42] These data indicate that the insulin-producing cells that result from in vitro differentiation have not progressed to fully matured, functional beta cells. Significantly, ESC-derived endocrine precursors, although multihormone positive, have the ability to form functional endocrine cells, including beta cells, when exposed to the appropriate in vivo–derived stimuli. Transplantation of ESC-derived endocrine precursors into immunocompromised severe combined immunodeficiency mice resulted in the final differentiation of beta cells and other hormone-secreting cells. These beta cells were functional because they were sufficient to restore euglycemia after chemical-induced diabetes with streptozotocin.[56] Removal of the transplanted cells resulted in a recurrence of hyperglycemia. These data support the hypothesis that ESC-derived cells are able to mature into function beta cells if exposed to the appropriate signals.

Although evidence of emerging beta cells has been observed in appropriately stimulated ESCs, it is unclear if functional islets can be formed by such in vitro approaches. In 2-dimensional culture, important pancreatic matrix cues are likely to be absent. In utero islets develop into 3-dimensional (3D) structures having interactions with epithelial cells. These signals are missing in culture. Moreover, cell-cell interactions between mesenchyme and other germ layers (mesoderm and ectoderm) are omitted in the relatively pure cell population that results from the specialized differentiation of ESCs to definitive endoderm. Islets are complex structures that consist of multiple cell types in an intricate orchestrated structure. In addition to hormone-secreting cells, neuronal and vascular endothelial cells are interlaced in the 3D islet structure, providing interactions both between and within cell types. These interactions seem to be essential for insulin sensing and secretion.[58] Alternate culture techniques might be required to facilitate appropriate interactions in deriving islets or functional beta cells from ESCs.

In addition to the significant challenge of appropriately nurturing ESCs to functional beta cells by providing commitment stimuli in the required temporal context at the desired concentration with an ordered 3D interactive environment, several key issues are associated with the clinical use of ESCs. Ethically, ESC research is a complex and highly emotive area.[59,60] Further, beta cells derived from ESCs present the risk of cancer formation. Transplantation of cells enriched in human ESC-derived pancreatic progenitors, when grafted in mice, was associated with teratoma formation.[56] In addition, ESCs are mismatched tissue and are subject to immune rejection. Immunosuppression to prevent allogeneic graft rejection, which carries the limitations outlined under the transplantation of donor islets, is likely to be required. In the setting of type 1 diabetes, host autoimmune rejection (which leads to the initial loss of beta cells) also needs suppression.

iPSC

Recent breakthroughs in cellular reprogramming have presented the potential of an alternative approach in stem cell technology, which may circumvent allogeneic immune rejection. The paradigm-changing studies arising from the laboratories of Thomson and Yamanaka demonstrated that a cocktail of only 4 different transcription factors is required to reprogram somatic cells into iPSCs. The iPSCs have characteristics similar to ESCs, such as the ability to retain unlimited self-renewal capacity[61,62] and differentiate into all 3 germ layers, the endoderm, mesoderm, and ectoderm. Although resetting the dogma, these exciting studies raise the potential that generation of patient-specific stem cell populations may become a feasible option.[61–64] These autologous cells may also circumvent the requirement for immunosuppression. The application of the initial studies to a clinical setting was limited because of the use of lentiviruses and retroviruses to force the introduction and expression of the transcription factors in somatic cells. Strategies to reprogram cells into iPSCs without the use of virus have recently been developed.[65–67] The question remains if iPSCs acquire the full capacity for differentiation associated with ESCs. Most recent studies in mice suggest that unlike ESCs, an important gene cluster located in a segment of chromosome 12 is shut off in iPSCs. This segment contains genes that are important for fetal development and is prohibitive to full development if silenced, as occurs in most iPSCs.[68] Should the iPSCs derived from human cells have similar differences in gene expression, additional and new reprogramming strategies may be required.

Although the clear future utility of ESC- or iPSC-derived islets depends on the elucidation of defined pharmacologic, temporal, and morphometric approaches to guide appropriate differentiation of pluripotent cells to beta cells and/or islets, the attraction of an unlimited cell source remains apparent.

REPROGRAMMING THE ADULT STEM CELL

Plasticity of the adult pancreas is recognized under conditions of pregnancy and obesity as an adaptive response to increased metabolic burden.[9] Implicit, therefore, is the concept of protodifferentiated cells residing in the pancreas, which are capable of dividing and expanding to generate new islet mass. Targeting an endogenous adult pancreatic stem cell offers several significant advantages over targeting an exogenous one (cell replacement strategies). These include

- Provides potential for pharmacologic manipulation
- Avoids requirement of systemic immunosuppression
- Eliminates risk of teratoma formation associated with pluripotent stem cells.

An adult pancreatic stem cell is a pancreatic protodifferentiated cell that retains the ability to differentiate, divide, dedifferentiate, or transdifferentiate to expand the beta-cell mass. The source of a pancreatic precursor cell has been keenly studied and hotly contested in recent years. Research indicates that there is more than one source of pancreatic stem cell or means of producing beta cells.

BETA CELLS FROM BETA CELLS

Regeneration, the creation of beta cells from the self-renewal of existing beta cells, has been proposed as a mechanism for increasing endogenous beta-cell mass. In the partial pancreatectomy model, using lineage-tracing studies, regrowth of beta cells was shown to derive mainly from the proliferation of existing beta cells.[69] The question of whether a specialized stem cell is present in the beta-cell pool or if all beta cells possess the propensity to proliferate has further been addressed. Beta cells appear to be homogenous in their ability to contribute to replication because no specialized subset of beta cells was identified in a variety of tracing techniques studied.[70,71] These studies have concluded that beta-cell replication is a primary source of facultative beta-cell mass expansion after partial pancreatectomy and during pregnancy. Beta-cell replication has also been suggested to be a primary mechanism in the postnatal expansion of beta-cell mass in human diabetes.[72] Turnover of adult beta cells is very low,[73] and regeneration from a beta-cell pool is a limited strategy in terms of diabetes therapy because the beta cells are likely to be defective or absent.

BETA CELLS FROM ACINAR CELLS

Transdifferentiation, the ability to switch the characteristics of a differentiated cell to a new cell type, has been described in the pancreas. Differentiated adult pancreatic exocrine cells were induced to dedifferentiate and subsequently redifferentiate to become like a beta cell.[74] Intriguingly, in a manner analogous to the conversion of adult cells into iPSCs, this conversion was achieved by just introducing 3 transcription factors (ngn3, Pdx1 and Mafa). Melton and colleagues[74] identified key signaling pathways associated with de- and redifferentiation from mouse exocrine cells. On reprogramming, acinar cells transdifferentiate to beta cells in isolation and do not form organized islet structures. Interestingly, these data revive the notion of an insulo-acinar transformation proposed by Lewaschew[75] in 1886 and progressed in the early nineteenth century before being superseded by better cell identification techniques.

BETA CELLS FROM ALPHA CELLS

Transdifferentiation between pancreatic cells has recently been revisited with the studies of Herrara and colleagues,[76] who reported the conversion of pancreatic alpha cells to beta cells under a condition of extreme beta-cell loss. The key feature of their study was the near-complete (98%) elimination of endogenous beta cells using a mild ablation technique. Beta cells were genetically engineered to be selectively sensitive to deletion using diphtheria toxin. Unlike other models, such as partial pancreatectomy, this approach induced the heterologous regeneration of beta cells from an alpha-cell source.

A key observation was that the program for alpha-cell differentiation was observed only when beta-cell mass was eliminated because alpha-cell transdifferentiation was not seen in hemizygous animals that had a 50% elimination of endogenous beta cells. This permissive pathway is likely to result from the release of some inhibitory signals, such as those mediated by the Pax4 and Arx axis. The ectopic expression of Pax4 in alpha cells results in the conversion of alpha cells to beta cells.[77]

These data also raise the notion that different programs are available to increase the beta-cell mass and that they are accessible depending on the degree of beta-cell loss. Beta-cell replication is seen in the partial pancreatectomy model and during pregnancy, in which there is significant beta-cell retention. Alpha-cell transdifferentiation was only observed when beta-cell mass was eliminated.

BETA CELLS FROM DUCT CELLS

Islet neogenesis refers to the differentiation of progenitor cells that reside in the pancreatic duct epithelium and give rise to islet cell types. This paradigm recapitulates islet development in utero in that it recreates endocrine cell development that arises during secondary transition. Partial ligation of the pancreatic duct stimulates adult islet neogenesis, a phenomenon first described in 1902 by Laguesse and de la Roche.[78] This model has been adapted to study islet neogenesis[79–83] and has provided compelling support for the plasticity of adult pancreatic duct cells to differentiate into functional endocrine cells. Most recently, Xu and colleagues[84] identified progenitor cells located in the ductal epithelium of the adult pancreas, which can be induced to develop into newly formed beta cells. Ligation of the duct leading to the pancreatic tail in BALB/c mice induced expression of ngn3 in the pancreatic duct, which accompanied a doubling in pancreatic beta-cell mass. Only the ligated part of the pancreas was affected. The role for ngn3 in this pathway was confirmed using an interfering RNA gene-knockdown approach that prevented the increase in beta-cell mass associated with duct ligation.

PHARMACOLOGIC EXPANSION OF ENDOGENOUS BETA-CELL MASS

Trophic factors have been identified that induce islet neogenesis. Several factors are being evaluated in human clinical trials and include islet neogenesis associated protein (INGAP), the stable analogues of the incretin glucagon-like peptide 1 (GLP-1), and the growth factor combination of epidermal growth factor (EGF) plus gastrin, termed I.N.T. therapy.

INGAP is a bioactive protein identified in the duct ligation model of islet neogenesis. INGAP or the bioactive INGAP peptide stimulates new islet growth when administered to rodents,[82,85,86] dogs,[87] or primates[88] as evidenced by an increase in beta-cell mass identified in quantitative histologic analyses and measurement of insulin levels. The increase in beta-cell mass was sufficient to reverse induced diabetes in mice.[82] Recent human studies of INGAP offer support that INGAP therapy could be clinically relevant. Results from these trials showed an approximate 1% reduction in HbA1c (a clinical marker of glucose exposure) in patients with type 2 diabetes and a statistical significant improvement in stimulated C peptide (a marker of insulin production) in patients with type 1 diabetes.[89] The action of INGAP in recapitulating the embryonic development program in the adult ductal precursor cell is supported in studies that describe INGAP immunoreactivity in the embryonic pancreas associated with a precursor endocrine cell[90] and a report of the differentiation of mouse ESCs to a beta-cell like phenotype after stimulation with INGAP.[91]

GLP-1 is a short-acting peptide hormone secreted from the gut in response to food ingestion. GLP-1 exerts a variety of important metabolic functions; in the brain, it promotes satiety and reduces appetite[92]; in the stomach, it regulates gastric emptying; and in the pancreas,[93] it reduces postprandial glucagon secretion in alpha cells[94] and enhances glucose-dependent insulin secretion in beta cells.[95] GLP-1 has been associated with the induction of islet neogenesis in the Goto-Kakizaki rat[96] and reversal of hyperglycemia in diabetic mice when combined with gastrin.[97] GLP-1, however, is rapidly degraded ($t_{1/2}<2$ minutes) by the ubiquitous peptidase, dipeptidyl peptidase-IV (DPP-IV). Accordingly, inhibitors of DPP-IV (eg, sitagliptin, saxagliptin, and vildagliptin) are potential indirect stimuli of endogenous pancreatic adult cells because of their ability to extend the biologic half-life of endogenous GLP-1. Exenatide is a synthetic stable analogue of GLP-1, which is resistant to DPP-IV protease activity. In transplant recipients that have islet graft dysfunction, the administration of a subsequent, supplemental, islet infusion when concurrent with exenatide treatment promoted long-term insulin independence to an extent greater than a supplemental islet infusion alone.[98] This action of exenatide is believed to be via an antiapoptotic mechanism of GLP-1, thereby protecting the infused islets. Stable GLP-1 has been incorporated in several ESC differentiation protocols to promote insulin secretion and to suppress apoptosis of pre–beta cells.

I.N.T. therapy has a focus on inducing islet neogenesis with a combination of EGF and a gastrin analog (G1) or GLP-1 and G1. EGF receptor signaling induces stimulation of fetal pancreatic ducts, and islet cell differentiation is delayed in mice lacking EGF receptors.[40] Gastrin is expressed during pancreas development at the point in which protodifferentiated ducts transform to form the fully differentiated exocrine and endocrine pancreas.[99] The combination of EGF and gastrin resulted in a 3-fold increase in beta-cell number in adult human pancreatic tissue cultures in vitro.[100] Islet neogenesis from pancreatic duct precursor cells is the mechanism behind this expansion in beta-cell mass, as shown in the combination of gastrin and GLP-1.[97,100]

SUMMARY

Restoring a functional beta-cell population for patients with diabetes is a prime focus in diabetes research. Islet and/or beta-cell transplantation, likely, has the shortest path to achieve clinical use, but it is also fraught with the most potential pitfalls, including ethical considerations, paucity of available donor islets, and complications associated with antirejection medications. Although solutions are being sought for these drawbacks, the possibility of repopulating the endocrine pancreas from precursor cells that are already resident in the pancreas is an exciting prospect for the therapy for diabetes. It seems that under special conditions and depending on the state of the endogenous beta-cell mass, many of the pancreatic cell types can be induced to form beta cells. Pharmacologic interventions are being developed, which promote the induction of islet regeneration in vivo. An important future consideration is whether the beta cells produced in vivo through regeneration have regulated expansion and provide physiologically controlled insulin secretion. The prospect for an effective treatment of both type 1 and type 2 diabetes is tantalizingly close; yet, there remain many challenges to be overcome to determine the best therapeutic approach to harness the pancreatic stem cell. It is an exciting time for diabetes research, with the prospect for a significant breakthrough in therapeutic paradigms being so tangibly close.

REFERENCES

1. Ryan EA, Lakey JR, Paty BW, et al. Successful islet transplantation: continued insulin reserve provides long-term glycemic control. Diabetes 2002;51(7): 2148–57.

2. Hainz U, Jürgens B, Heitger A. The role of indoleamine 2,3-dioxygenase in transplantation. Transpl Int 2007;20(2):118–27.

3. Itakura S, Asari S, Rawson J, et al. Mesenchymal stem cells facilitate the induction of mixed hematopoietic chimerism and islet allograft tolerance without GVHD in the rat. Am J Transplant 2007;7(2):336–46.

4. Rehman KK, Bertera S, Trucco M, et al. Immunomodulation by adenoviral-mediated SCD40-Ig gene therapy for mouse allogeneic islet transplantation. Transplantation 2007;84(3):301–7.

5. Yang SH, Jin JZ, Lee SH, et al. Role of NKT cells in allogeneic islet graft survival. Clin Immunol 2007;124(3):258–66.

6. Pileggi A, Molano RD, Ricordi C, et al. Reversal of diabetes by pancreatic islet transplantation into a subcutaneous, neovascularized device. Transplantation 2006;81(9):1318–24.

7. Beck J, Angus R, Madsen B, et al. Islet encapsulation: strategies to enhance islet cell functions. Tissue Eng 2007;13(3):589–99.

8. Hirshberg B, Rother KI, Harlan DM. Islet transplantation: where do we stand now? Diabetes Metab Res Rev 2003;19(3):175–8 [discussion: 175].

9. Butler PC, Meier JJ, Butler AE, et al. The replication of beta cells in normal physiology, in disease and for therapy. Nat Clin Pract Endocrinol Metab 2007;3(11): 758–68.

10. Murtaugh LC, Melton DA. Genes, signals, and lineages in pancreas development. Annu Rev Cell Dev Biol 2003;19:71–89.

11. Apelqvist A, Ahlgren U, Edlund H. Sonic Hedgehog directs specialised mesoderm differentiation in the intestine and pancreas. Curr Biol 1997;7(10):801–4.

12. Hebrok M, Kim SK, Melton DA. Notochord repression of endodermal Sonic hedgehog permits pancreas development. Genes Dev 1998;12(11):1705–13.

13. Edlund H. Transcribing pancreas. Diabetes 1998;47(12):1817–23.

14. Kim SK, Hebrok M. Intercellular signals regulating pancreas development and function. Genes Dev 2001;15(2):111–27.

15. Kim SK, Hebrok M, Melton DA. Notochord to endoderm signaling is required for pancreas development. Development 1997;124(21):4243–52.

16. Kim W, Shin YK, Kim BJ, et al. Notch signaling in pancreatic endocrine cell and diabetes. Biochem Biophys Res Commun 2010;392(3):247–51.

17. Apelqvist A, Li H, Sommer L, et al. Notch signalling controls pancreatic cell differentiation. Nature 1999;400(6747):877–81.

18. Gradwohl G, Dierich A, LeMeur M, et al. Neurogenin3 is required for the development of the four endocrine cell lineages of the pancreas. Proc Natl Acad Sci U S A 2000;97(4):1607–11.

19. Gu G, Dubauskaite J, Melton DA. Direct evidence for the pancreatic lineage: Ngn3+ cells are islet progenitors and are distinct from duct progenitors. Development 2002;129(10):2447–57.

20. Schwitzgebel VM, Scheel DW, Conners JR, et al. Expression of neurogenin3 reveals an islet cell precursor population in the pancreas. Development 2000; 127(16):3533–42.

21. Herrera PL. Adult insulin- and glucagon-producing cells differentiate from two independent cell lineages. Development 2000;127(11):2317–22.

22. Herrera PL, Huarte J, Zufferey R, et al. Ablation of islet endocrine cells by targeted expression of hormone-promoter-driven toxigenes. Proc Natl Acad Sci U S A 1994;91(26):12999–3003.

23. Lee YC, Damholt AB, Billestrup N, et al. Developmental expression of proprotein convertase 1/3 in the rat. Mol Cell Endocrinol 1999;155(1–2):27–35.

24. Wilson ME, Kalamaras JA, German MS. Expression pattern of IAPP and prohormone convertase 1/3 reveals a distinctive set of endocrine cells in the embryonic pancreas. Mech Dev 2002;115(1–2):171–6.

25. Guney MA, Gannon M. Pancreas cell fate. Birth Defects Res C Embryo Today 2009;87(3):232–48.

26. Collombat P, Hecksher-Sorensen J, Broccoli V, et al. The simultaneous loss of ARX and PAX4 genes promotes a somatostatin-producing cell fate specification at the expense of the alpha- and beta-cell lineages in the mouse endocrine pancreas. Development 2005;132(13):2969–80.

27. Collombat P, Hecksher-Sorensen J, Krull J, et al. Embryonic endocrine pancreas and mature beta cells acquire alpha and pp cell phenotypes upon ARX misexpression. J Clin Invest 2007;117(4):961–70.

28. Collombat P, Mansouri A, Hecksher-Sorensen J, et al. Opposing actions of ARX and PAX4 in endocrine pancreas development. Genes Dev 2003;17(20):2591–603.

29. Ritz-Laser B, Estreicher A, Gauthier BR, et al. The pancreatic beta-cell-specific transcription factor PAX-4 inhibits glucagon gene expression through PAX-6. Diabetologia 2002;45(1):97–107.

30. Wang Q, Elghazi L, Martin S, et al. Ghrelin is a novel target of PAX4 in endocrine progenitors of the pancreas and duodenum. Dev Dyn 2008;237(1):51–61.

31. Sussel L, Kalamaras J, Hartigan-O'Connor DJ, et al. Mice lacking the homeodomain transcription factor Nkx2.2 have diabetes due to arrested differentiation of pancreatic beta cells. Development 1998;125(12):2213–21.

32. Fujimoto K, Polonsky KS. Pdx1 and other factors that regulate pancreatic beta-cell survival. Diabetes Obes Metab 2009;11(Suppl 4):30–7.

33. Taylor-Fishwick DA, Shi W, Pittenger GL, et al. Pdx-1 can repress stimulus-induced activation of the ingap promoter. J Endocrinol 2006;188(3):611–21.

34. Ahlgren U, Jonsson J, Jonsson L, et al. Beta-cell-specific inactivation of the mouse ipf1/pdx1 gene results in loss of the beta-cell phenotype and maturity onset diabetes. Genes Dev 1998;12(12):1763–8.

35. Dutta S, Bonner-Weir S, Montminy M, et al. Regulatory factor linked to late-onset diabetes? Nature 1998;392(6676):560.

36. Stoffers DA, Stanojevic V, Habener JF. Insulin promoter factor-1 gene mutation linked to early-onset type 2 diabetes mellitus directs expression of a dominant negative isoprotein. J Clin Invest 1998;102(1):232–41.

37. Ohneda K, Mirmira RG, Wang J, et al. The homeodomain of pdx-1 mediates multiple protein-protein interactions in the formation of a transcriptional activation complex on the insulin promoter. Mol Cell Biol 2000;20(3):900–11.

38. Gannon M, Ables ET, Crawford L, et al. Pdx-1 function is specifically required in embryonic beta cells to generate appropriate numbers of endocrine cell types and maintain glucose homeostasis. Dev Biol 2008;314(2):406–17.

39. Johansson KA, Dursun U, Jordan N, et al. Temporal control of neurogenin3 activity in pancreas progenitors reveals competence windows for the generation of different endocrine cell types. Dev Cell 2007;12(3):457–65.

40. Mimeault M, Hauke R, Batra SK. Stem cells: a revolution in therapeutics-recent advances in stem cell biology and their therapeutic applications in regenerative medicine and cancer therapies. Clin Pharmacol Ther 2007;82(3):252–64.

41. Assady S, Maor G, Amit M, et al. Insulin production by human embryonic stem cells. Diabetes 2001;50(8):1691–7.

42. D'Amour KA, Bang AG, Eliazer S, et al. Production of pancreatic hormone-expressing endocrine cells from human embryonic stem cells. Nat Biotechnol 2006;24(11):1392–401.

43. Segev H, Fishman B, Ziskind A, et al. Differentiation of human embryonic stem cells into insulin-producing clusters. Stem Cells 2004;22(3):265–74.

44. Lumelsky N, Blondel O, Laeng P, et al. Differentiation of embryonic stem cells to insulin-secreting structures similar to pancreatic islets. Science 2001;292(5520): 1389–94.

45. Hori Y, Rulifson IC, Tsai BC, et al. Growth inhibitors promote differentiation of insulin-producing tissue from embryonic stem cells. Proc Natl Acad Sci U S A 2002;99(25):16105–10.

46. Hansson M, Tonning A, Frandsen U, et al. Artifactual insulin release from differentiated embryonic stem cells. Diabetes 2004;53(10):2603–9.

47. Rajagopal J, Anderson WJ, Kume S, et al. Insulin staining of ES cell progeny from insulin uptake. Science 2003;299(5605):363.

48. Blyszczuk P, Czyz J, Kania G, et al. Expression of Pax4 in embryonic stem cells promotes differentiation of nestin-positive progenitor and insulin-producing cells. Proc Natl Acad Sci U S A 2003;100(3):998–1003.

49. Lavon N, Yanuka O, Benvenisty N. The effect of overexpression of Pdx1 and Foxa2 on the differentiation of human embryonic stem cells into pancreatic cells. Stem Cells 2006;24(8):1923–30.

50. Miyazaki S, Yamato E, Miyazaki J. Regulated expression of Pdx-1 promotes in vitro differentiation of insulin-producing cells from embryonic stem cells. Diabetes 2004;53(4):1030–7.

51. Treff NR, Vincent RK, Budde ML, et al. Differentiation of embryonic stem cells conditionally expressing neurogenin 3. Stem Cells 2006;24(11):2529–37.

52. Oliver-Krasinski JM, Stoffers DA. On the origin of the beta cell. Genes Dev 2008; 22(15):1998–2021.

53. Phillips BW, Hentze H, Rust WL, et al. Directed differentiation of human embryonic stem cells into the pancreatic endocrine lineage. Stem Cells Dev 2007; 16(4):561–78.

54. Jiang J, Au M, Lu K, et al. Generation of insulin-producing islet-like clusters from human embryonic stem cells. Stem Cells 2007;25(8):1940–53.

55. D'Amour KA, Agulnick AD, Eliazer S, et al. Efficient differentiation of human embryonic stem cells to definitive endoderm. Nat Biotechnol 2005;23(12): 1534–41.

56. Kroon E, Martinson LA, Kadoya K, et al. Pancreatic endoderm derived from human embryonic stem cells generates glucose-responsive insulin-secreting cells in vivo. Nat Biotechnol 2008;26(4):443–52.

57. Yao S, Chen S, Clark J, et al. Long-term self-renewal and directed differentiation of human embryonic stem cells in chemically defined conditions. Proc Natl Acad Sci U S A 2006;103(18):6907–12.

58. Ballian N, Brunicardi FC. Islet vasculature as a regulator of endocrine pancreas function. World J Surg 2007;31(4):705–14.

59. Green RM. Can we develop ethically universal embryonic stem-cell lines? Nat Rev Genet 2007;8(6):480–5.

60. Mauron A, Jaconi ME. Stem cell science: current ethical and policy issues. Clin Pharmacol Ther 2007;82(3):330–3.

61. Takahashi K, Tanabe K, Ohnuki M, et al. Induction of pluripotent stem cells from adult human fibroblasts by defined factors. Cell 2007;131(5):861–72.

62. Yu J, Vodyanik MA, Smuga-Otto K, et al. Induced pluripotent stem cell lines derived from human somatic cells. Science 2007;318(5858):1917–20.

63. Meissner A, Wernig M, Jaenisch R. Direct reprogramming of genetically unmodified fibroblasts into pluripotent stem cells. Nat Biotechnol 2007;25(10):1177–81.

64. Park IH, Zhao R, West JA, et al. Reprogramming of human somatic cells to pluripotency with defined factors. Nature 2008;451(7175):141–6.
65. Kaji K, Norrby K, Paca A, et al. Virus-free induction of pluripotency and subsequent excision of reprogramming factors. Nature 2009;458(7239):771–5.
66. Lin T, Ambasudhan R, Yuan X, et al. A chemical platform for improved induction of human ipscs. Nat Methods 2009;6(11):805–8.
67. Woltjen K, Michael IP, Mohseni P, et al. Piggybac transposition reprograms fibroblasts to induced pluripotent stem cells. Nature 2009;458(7239):766–70.
68. Stadtfeld M, Apostolou E, Akutsu H, et al. Aberrant silencing of imprinted genes on chromosome 12qF1 in mouse induced pluripotent stem cells. Nature 2010; 465(7295):175–81.
69. Dor Y, Brown J, Martinez OI, et al. Adult pancreatic beta-cells are formed by self-duplication rather than stem-cell differentiation. Nature 2004;429(6987): 41–6.
70. Brennand K, Huangfu D, Melton D. All beta cells contribute equally to islet growth and maintenance. PLoS Biol 2007;5(7):e163.
71. Teta M, Rankin MM, Long SY, et al. Growth and regeneration of adult beta cells does not involve specialized progenitors. Dev Cell 2007;12(5):817–26.
72. Meier JJ, Butler AE, Saisho Y, et al. Beta-cell replication is the primary mechanism subserving the postnatal expansion of beta-cell mass in humans. Diabetes 2008;57(6):1584–94.
73. Teta M, Long SY, Wartschow LM, et al. Very slow turnover of beta-cells in aged adult mice. Diabetes 2005;54(9):2557–67.
74. Zhou Q, Brown J, Kanarek A, et al. In vivo reprogramming of adult pancreatic exocrine cells to beta-cells. Nature 2008;455(7213):627–32.
75. Lewaschew SW. Ueber eine eigenthiimliche Verinderung des Pancreaszellen warmbliutiger Thiere bei starker absonderungs- thiitigkeit der Driise. Archiv f Mikero Anat 1885;Bd.26,s:453–85.
76. Thorel F, Nepote V, Avril I, et al. Conversion of adult pancreatic alpha-cells to beta-cells after extreme beta-cell loss. Nature 2010;464(7292):1149–54.
77. Collombat P, Xu X, Ravassard P, et al. The ectopic expression of pax4 in the mouse pancreas converts progenitor cells into alpha and subsequently beta cells. Cell 2009;138(3):449–62.
78. Laguesse E, de la Roche AG. Les ilots de langerhans dans le pancreas du cobaye après ligature. C R Seances Soc Biol 1902;54:854–7 [in French].
79. Bonner-Weir S, Inada A, Yatoh S, et al. Transdifferentiation of pancreatic ductal cells to endocrine beta-cells. Biochem Soc Trans 2008;36(Pt 3):353–6.
80. Li M, Miyagawa J, Yamamoto K, et al. Beta cell neogenesis from ducts and phenotypic conversion of residual islet cells in the adult pancreas of glucose intolerant mice induced by selective alloxan perfusion. Endocrinol Jpn 2002; 49(5):561–72.
81. Pittenger GL, Taylor-Fishwick DA, Vinik AI. A role for islet neogenesis in curing diabetes. Diabetologia, 2009;52(5):735–8.
82. Rosenberg L, Lipsett M, Yoon JW, et al. A pentadecapeptide fragment of islet neogenesis-associated protein increases beta-cell mass and reverses diabetes in C57bl/6j mice. Ann Surg 2004;240(5):875–84.
83. Vinik AI, Rosenberg L, Pittenger GL, et al. Stimulation of pancreatic islet neogenesis: a possible treatment for type 1 and type 2 diabetes. Curr Opin Endocrinol Diabetes 2004;11:125–40.
84. Xu X, D'Hoker J, Stange G, et al. Beta cells can be generated from endogenous progenitors in injured adult mouse pancreas. Cell 2008;132(2):197–207.

85. Rosenberg L, Vinik AI, Pittenger GL, et al. Islet-cell regeneration in the diabetic hamster pancreas with restoration of normoglycaemia can be induced by a local growth factor(s). Diabetologia 1996;39(3):256–62.

86. Taylor-Fishwick DA, Bowman A, Hamblet N, et al. Islet neogenesis associated protein transgenic mice are resistant to hyperglycemia induced by streptozotocin. J Endocrinol 2006;190(3):729–37.

87. Pittenger GL, Taylor-Fishwick DA, Johns RH, et al. Intramuscular injection of islet neogenesis-associated protein peptide stimulates pancreatic islet neogenesis in healthy dogs. Pancreas 2007;34(1):103–11.

88. Fleming A, Rosenberg L. Prospects and challenges for islet regeneration as a treatment for diabetes: a review of islet neogenesis associated protein. J Diabetes Sci Tech 2007;1:231–44.

89. Dungan KM, Buse JB, Ratner RE. Effects of therapy in type 1 and type 2 diabetes mellitus with a peptide derived from islet neogenesis associated protein (INGAP). Diabetes Metab Res Rev 2009;25(6):558–65.

90. Hamblet NS, Shi W, Vinik AI, et al. The reg family member ingap is a marker of endocrine patterning in the embryonic pancreas. Pancreas 2008;36(1):1–9.

91. Francini F, Del Zotto H, Massa ML, et al. Selective effect of ingap-pp upon mouse embryonic stem cell differentiation toward islet cells. Regul Pept 2009; 153(1–3):43–8.

92. Flint A, Raben A, Astrup A, et al. Glucagon-like peptide 1 promotes satiety and suppresses energy intake in humans. J Clin Invest 1998;101(3):515–20.

93. Nauck MA, Wollschlager D, Werner J, et al. Effects of subcutaneous glucagon-like peptide 1 (glp-1 [7–36 amide]) in patients with niddm. Diabetologia 1996; 39(12):1546–53.

94. Larsson H, Holst JJ, Ahren B. Glucagon-like peptide-1 reduces hepatic glucose production indirectly through insulin and glucagon in humans. Acta Physiol Scand 1997;160(4):413–22.

95. Drucker DJ. Glucagon-like peptides. Diabetes 1998;47(2):159–69.

96. Tourrel C, Bailbe D, Lacorne M, et al. Persistent improvement of type 2 diabetes in the goto-kakizaki rat model by expansion of the beta-cell mass during the prediabetic period with glucagon-like peptide-1 or exendin-4. Diabetes 2002; 51(5):1443–52.

97. Brand SJ, Tagerud S, Lambert P, et al. Pharmacological treatment of chronic diabetes by stimulating pancreatic beta-cell regeneration with systemic co-administration of EGF and gastrin. Pharmacol Toxicol 2002;91(6):414–20.

98. Ghofaili KA, Fung M, Ao Z, et al. Effect of exenatide on beta cell function after islet transplantation in type 1 diabetes. Transplantation 2007;83(1):24–8.

99. Brand SJ, Fuller PJ. Differential gastrin gene expression in rat gastrointestinal tract and pancreas during neonatal development. J Biol Chem 1988;263(11): 5341–7.

100. Suarez-Pinzon WL, Lakey JR, Brand SJ, et al. Combination therapy with epidermal growth factor and gastrin induces neogenesis of human islet {beta}-cells from pancreatic duct cells and an increase in functional {beta}-cell mass. J Clin Endocrinol Metab 2005;90(6):3401–9.

Circulating Biomarkers in Neuroendocrine Tumors of the Enteropancreatic Tract: Application to Diagnosis, Monitoring Disease, and as Prognostic Indicators

Joy E.S. Ardill, PhD, MRCPath[a], Thomas M. O'Dorisio, MD[b],*

KEYWORDS

- Neuroendocrine tumors • Prognostic indicators
- Circulating biomarkers • Disease monitoring

Neuroendocrine tumors (NETs) are difficult to diagnose. Their symptoms may be vague or intermittent, and are frequently associated with much more common diseases; many of the tumors may be asymptomatic. Therefore, diagnosis can be delayed for some years. Because most NETs are secretory, the measurement of circulating biomarkers is helpful not only for diagnosis but also for assessing tumor response to treatment, monitoring disease progression, and use as prognostic indicators.

Three technologies are used in the diagnosis of NETs: radiology, measurement of circulating tumor biomarkers, and tissue pathology. Each has advantages and disadvantages. Radiology (computed tomography [CT] and magnetic resonance imaging [MRI]) offers visualization, but only for lesions greater than 1.5 cm in diameter and, as many NETs are small (or both small and multiple) this technique has limitations. Liver and lymphatic metastases may be numerous but small resulting in an inability to assess metastatic spread at an early stage. In addition, radiological procedures are costly when used for frequent follow-up and in the cases of CT scans and somatostatin analogue scintigraphy or fluorodeoxyglucose (FDG)-positron emission tomography (PET) scans, accumulative

[a] Regional Regulatory Peptide Laboratory, Kelvin Building, Royal Victoria Hospital, Grosvenor Road, Belfast, BT 126BA, UK
[b] Department of Internal Medicine, Division of Endocrinology/Metabolism/Diabetes, University of Iowa Hospitals & Clinics, Iowa City, IA, USA
* Corresponding author.
E-mail address: thomas-odorisio@uiowa.edu

Endocrinol Metab Clin N Am 39 (2010) 777–790
doi:10.1016/j.ecl.2010.09.001
0889-8529/10/$ – see front matter © 2010 Published by Elsevier Inc.
endo.theclinics.com

radiation dose must be taken into consideration, particularly for the younger patient. Although radiological procedures are less sensitive than measurements of circulating tumor biomarkers or actual tissue pathology, they remain the gold standard by which therapeutic interventions are determined. Measurement of circulating biomarkers is noninvasive and relatively inexpensive but there are significant problems with false-positive results. Because of this, it is less useful as a diagnostic tool but much more useful for following disease progression and treatment and as a prognostic indicator.

Tissue pathology offers the definitive diagnosis and proliferative index from a needle biopsy or surgical specimen. The limitation is that this gives 1 time point only in the disease pathway and repeat specimens are usually difficult to justify clinically. In addition, there is concern that a specimen may not be representative of the whole tumor, or 1 metastatic deposit may be quite different to another or to the primary tumor.

Therefore, the 3 technologies are complementary for diagnosis but the measurement of circulating biomarkers is most informative when used after the initial diagnosis has been made.[1]

LABORATORY DIAGNOSIS OF NETs: USING CIRCULATING TUMOR BIOMARKERS
General Biomarkers

There are several families of secretory proteins found in high concentrations in neuroendocrine cells and, in particular, neuroendocrine tumor cells. These proteins are used in the identification of NETs in the pathology laboratory. They include the granins, neurone-specific enolase (NSE), and synaptophysin. Both chromogranin A (CgA) and NSE are found in increased concentrations in the circulation of many patients with NETs and both have been used as general biomarkers for these tumors. CgA is well established as the most sensitive, indeed only general biomarker for NETs[2] and has been investigated extensively.[3–6] In normal physiology, most CgA found in the circulation is derived from enterocromaffin-like (ECL) cells in the stomach, but in patients with NETs, the main source is the tumor itself and the level of CgA in the circulation may be increased as much as 300-fold. The level of CgA is not increased in patients with benign NETs, which include almost all appendiceal NETs, most insulinomas (75%), many pulmonary NETs, and a significant number of NETs in the duodenum and rectum. CgA may not be increased in patients with multiple endocrine neoplasia type 1 (MEN1) or in patients with poorly differentiated NETs. Therefore, CgA is not a universal biomarker for NETs.

Circulating CgA is increased in several common conditions, notable when there is little or no acid in the stomach. This includes patients with atrophic gastritis and those who are chronically treated with proton pump inhibitor (PPI) drugs. This is a significant proportion of the adult population. When gastric acid is absent, the negative feedback to gastrin is absent. Therefore, gastrin continues to be stimulated. This increased amount of gastrin in turn stimulates the ECL cell to secrete CgA. Therefore, CgA increases in the circulation.

CgA is also increased in patients with renal impairment when CgA cannot be cleared from the circulation. Therefore, false-positives in CgA assays are a significant problem. Many false-positives occur in the range 2 to 4 times the reference range but a significant number also occur in the range 5 to 20 times the reference range. Less than 1% of CgA tests that are more than 20 times greater than the reference range are false-positives. **Fig. 1** shows circulating CgA concentrations in 12 individuals who were being treated with PPIs and following withdrawal of the drug.

Eight of 12 patients returned to normal within 7 days.[7] The longer they are on PPIs (especially the higher potency PPIs), the longer it takes the CgAs to normalize. This may be weeks.

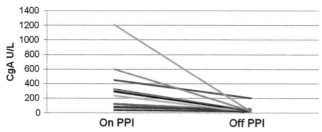

Fig. 1. Circulating CgA in patients on PPI and after withdrawal (N = 12). Reference range for CgA less than 30 units/L.

CgA has 439 amino acid residues with 11 pairs of dibasic residues and undergoes posttranslational processing that generates several products. Many of these products have been studied with respect to their potential as circulating biomarkers for NETs. The most interesting, clinically, is pancreastatin. Before the sequence of CgA was known and before there were any reliable assays that could measure the whole molecule, pancreastatin was used as a surrogate biomarker for CgA and was found to be significantly increased in the circulation of patients with NETs that had metastasized to liver. In some laboratories, pancreastatin measurement is preferred to whole molecule CgA measurement for the diagnosis and monitoring of NETs. Assays that measure midmolecule pancreastatin tend to cross-react strongly with CgA, whereas assays that detect the free C- or N-terminals of pancreastatin measure only this processed molecule; these assays are more interesting and have been recently shown to be clinically relevant.[8,9] Pancreastatin is not increased in patients with gastric achlorhydria or hypochlorhydria as posttranslational processing of CgA differs in tumor patients. Therefore, false-positives are less problematic with the pancreastatin assay. It may well prove to be a very early biomarker for liver tumor activity, even when CgA is in the normal range.

Chromogranin B (CgB) is the second granin that has undergone investigation. It has 14 dibasic cleavage points but has been less well studied than CgA. CgB circulates in much lower concentrations than does CgA in most patients with NETs. However, in tumors where CgA is not found, CgB may be increased.[10] Such patients include those with MEN1 and those with tumors in the duodenum or rectum. In these groups, CgB measurement may be useful.

SPECIFIC TUMOR BIOMARKERS FOR NETs OF PANCREATIC ORIGIN

About 6.5% of NETs occur in the pancreas. They may be benign or malignant and 15% to 20% are linked to an autosomal dominant gene mutation on chromosome 11 in MEN1.[11]

The most common secretory NET of the pancreas that produces a symptomatic complex is insulinoma. More than 80% of insulinomas are benign. Insulinoma is uncommon in MEN1 although it is the second most common pancreatic NET to occur in patients with MEN1. Insulinomas secrete proinsulin, insulin and C-peptide intermittently, and, although insulin concentrations in the circulation may often be within reference range, insulin is at most times inappropriately high for the blood glucose concentration. Patients present with the symptoms associated with symptomatic hypoglycemia (palpations, sweating pallor, anxiety, personality changes, and loss of consciousness). The latter symptom reflects both the severity and duration of hypoglycemia (see article elsewhere in this issue). Although these symptoms are profound, they may be intermittent and diagnosis is not always straightforward. A carefully supervised 72-hour starvation usually precipitates hypoglycemia within the first 36 to 48 hours. The differential diagnosis is insulin abuse (eg, known insulin-requiring diabetes or factitious hypoglycemia), which is uncommon. With insulin abuse, circulating insulin is increased but not proinsulin or C-peptide, so the measurement of increased proinsulin or C-peptide secures the diagnosis of insulinoma.[12] On rare occasions, patients treated with oral hypoglycemic medication (sulfonylureas) in the setting of renal compromise may show symptoms that mimic insulinoma. As most insulinomas are benign, CgA in not increased in this population. However, CgA measurement can be a useful indicator of malignancy in insulinoma.

Gastrinoma is the second most common secretory pancreatic NET with just more than half malignant at presentation. Approximately 25% to 35% of gastrinomas are associated with MEN1. Gastrinoma is the most common gastroenteropancreatic tumor associated with MEN1. Gastrinomas secrete gastrin but, because gastrin circulates in numerous forms, this is not exclusively gastrin 17. Progastrin, gastrin 34, gastrin 17, and C-terminally extended gastrins may all circulate in high concentrations in patients with gastrinoma. Patients usually present with hyperchlorhydria, which results in peptic ulceration that may extend throughout the stomach, the duodenum, and into the jejunum. When untreated, this results in severe pain and hematemesis. Before the development of acid-controlling drugs, gastrinoma was a life-threatening disease. Since the advent of H2 antagonists and PPIs, the syndrome is controlled by these drugs in the early stages, which results in a delayed diagnosis. Suspicion of gastrinoma should be raised with any patient who has recurrent ulcer in the absence of *Helicobactor pylori* infection. In addition to gastrin and CgA, pancreatic polypeptide (PP) may be increased in 35% to 40% of patients with gastrinoma. The increase in circulating gastrin may be small. In 20% of cases, circulating gastrin may be only 5% to 20% more than the reference range at presentation.[13] This is particularly evident when gastrin 17 and gastrin 34 are the predominant products secreted, as acid secretion is powerfully stimulated and severe symptoms develop rapidly.

The diagnosis of gastrinoma is not without difficulty in the laboratory. All patients with peptic ulcer symptoms receive acid-suppressing therapy, usually PPIs. In any patient receiving PPIs, both gastrin and CgA are increased to within the range of that recorded in many patients with gastrinoma.[14] When the negative feedback of acid is absent because of acid-suppressing therapy, gastrin and CgA continue to be stimulated and circulating concentrations of these cell products increase. This is also true for patients with atrophic gastritis. In patients in whom there is a suspicion of gastrinoma, PPIs should be withdrawn under careful supervision, as hematemesis and perforation may be a significant risk. A fasting blood specimen taken 5 to 7 days after withdrawal of PPI therapy will show a significant reduction in circulating gastrin and CgA in patients who do not have gastrinoma. In patients not on PPIs, autoimmune atrophic gastritis must also be excluded. Even considering the problems associated with the laboratory diagnosis of gastrinoma, the measurement of gastrin and CgA remains important in these patients.

Gastrinomas may be small and multiple, smaller than can be visualized by any current radiological method. Therefore, circulating gastrin remains a useful tool for diagnosis. Because of the problems associated with multiple small lesions in the pancreas for both gastrinoma and insulinoma, intraoperative venous sampling with rapid assay for the relevant peptides may be helpful to ensure that adequate surgery has been performed.

In addition, the secretin stimulation test may be used for the diagnosis of gastrinoma. Highly purified porcine secretion (2 units/kg body weight bolus) remains the best test for detecting the existence of gastrinoma. A paradoxic release of gastrin of 200 pg/mL from basal is diagnostic for the presence of gastrinoma in more than 90% of cases.[15]

VIPoma is much less common that insulinoma and gastrinoma with an incidence of approximately 0.02 per 100,000 per year. VIPoma is characterized by watery diarrhea, hypokalemia and achlorhydria (WDHA syndrome). The clinical features are caused by vasoactive intestinal peptide (VIP), which is a potent stimulator of intestinal secretion and inhibitor of gastric acid secretion. Diarrhea maybe watery and may escalate to 15 to 20 L per day causing the control of fluid and electrolytes (especially K^+ and HCO_3^-) to be critically compromised. Relatively small chronic increases in VIP in the circulation result in a profound VIPoma syndrome and patients frequently present when circulating VIP is no more than 20% to 50% more than the reference range. VIP acts as a neuromodulator and not a hormone in normal physiology; thus, it circulates in low quantities unless associated with a pathologic condition as seen in VIP-secreting NETs. There are several excellent VIP assays available in Europe and the United States.

Glucagonoma occurs at approximately the same frequency as VIPoma. In normal physiologic conditions, glucagon and its associated gene products are secreted from the alpha cells of the islets of Langerhans and from the L cells in the intestinal mucosa. From these 2 sites, proglucagon is processed differently. In the pancreas, proglucagon is processed to produce glucagon, glycentin-related peptide, intervening peptide, and the major glucagon fragment. Intestinal proglucagon undergoes alternative posttranslational processing that generates glycentin, sometimes referred to as gut glucagon, glucagon-like peptide 1 (GLP1), and glucagon-like peptide 2 (GLP2). Glycentin contains the glucagon sequence but is extended at the C-terminus.[16] Considering the importance of glucagon in the control of blood glucose one would expect a glucagon-secreting tumor to produce a profound syndrome. However this is not the case and glucagonoma usually presents late with extensive metastatic spread, mild diabetes, and a characteristic rash (necrolytic migratory erythema). Circulating glucagon concentrations are typically more than 5-fold higher than the reference range. Both pancreatic glucagon and glycentin are measured in high concentrations. When the tumor products are processed according to the pattern seen in the intestinal cells, then GLP1 and/or GLP2 may also be significantly increased. When secreted under tumor conditions, GLP2 results in the development of giant intestinal villi. In glucagon-secreting tumors, the measurement of CgA, glucagon, glycentin, GLP1, and GLP2 may be helpful. Although pancreatic glucagon measurements are readily obtainable in Europe and the United States, GLP1 is more difficult to obtain commercially. An excellent GLP1 radioimmunoassay is available in Denmark.[17]

Pancreatic somatostatinoma is uncommon and symptoms are vague thus diagnosis is frequently delayed. Patients may present with mild diabetes and steatorrhoea but more frequently with symptoms associated with tumor bulk. Circulating somatostatin concentrations may be more than 100 times the reference range.

PP-secreting pancreatic tumors are not associated with clinical signs and remain undetected in the early stages, becoming apparent because of symptoms associated with tumor bulk as disease progresses, or as an incidental finding. At the time of diagnosis, circulating PP may be more than 100 times higher than the reference range.

CgA is also increased in patients with glucagonoma, VIPoma, somatostatinoma, and PPoma when disease is metastatic, which is usual at diagnosis. In a significant number of patients with a pancreatic NET (35%), PP may be raised in addition to the specific syndrome tumor biomarker (**Table 1**).[1]

Table 1
Specific biomarkers for pancreatic NETs

Tumor Type	Syndrome	Symptoms	Circulating Biomarkers
Insulinoma	Whipple's triad	Hypoglycemia, dizziness, sweating	CgA and CgB, insulin inappropriate for blood glucose level, proinsulin, C-peptide
Gastrinoma	Zollinger-Ellison	Epigastric pain, peptic ulcer, diarrhea	CgA, gastrin, PP (35%)
VIPoma	WDHA	Watery diarrhea	CgA, VIP
Glucagonoma	None	NME	CgA, glucagon, glycentin
Somatostatinoma	None	Mild diabetes	CgA, somatostatin
PPoma	None	None	CgA, PP
Nonsecreting	None	None	CgA

CgA is raised only in metastatic tumors.
Abbreviations: NME, necrolytic migratory erythema; WDHA, watery diarrhea hypokalemia, and achlorhydria.

A significant number of pancreatic NETs are termed nonsecretory because they do not secrete any peptide or it may be that they secrete 1 or several peptides that do not cause observed imbalance to normal physiology and as yet these potential biomarkers have not been identified. These tumors normally secrete CgA when they are malignant.

Patients with MEN1 possess the potential to produce several different tumors of endocrine origin including the potential of these tumors to change tumor cell type. Commonly in the pancreas, a tumor that secretes 1 peptide progresses to the situation where there are some cells, clusters of cells or indeed discrete tumors develop that produce other peptides. Similarly, in malignant sporadic pancreatic NETs, the same potential exists and may be manifest in 50% of patients with metastatic gastrinoma. In sporadic pancreatic NETs, this is associated with a worsening prognosis, and with the secretion of some products such as adrenocorticotropic hormone (ACTH), the prognosis becomes very poor.[18] Early identification of any such change is important as more aggressive treatment options must be followed promptly. A regular annual screen for a variety of these circulating biomarkers is recommended for both patients with MEN1 and those with sporadic metastatic pancreatic NETs. This should include insulin, gastrin, VIP, glucagon, somatostatin, PP, calcitonin, prolactin, and ACTH (**Fig. 2**).

Simple tumors secrete gastrin only. Complex tumors may begin as simple gastrinomas but progress, secreting additional peptides including glucagon, insulin VIP, calcitonin, somatostatin prolactin, and ACTH.

SPECIFIC BIOMARKERS OF NETS OF GASTROINTESTINAL ORIGIN
Stomach

There are 3 types of NETs that occur in the stomach, and the incidence of these tumors is much higher than was believed some years ago.

Type 1 is associated with atrophic gastritis and is related to the absence of negative feedback resulting from the achlorhydric stomach. Increased gastrin in the circulation continuously drives the ECL cell resulting in the development of ECL adenomas.

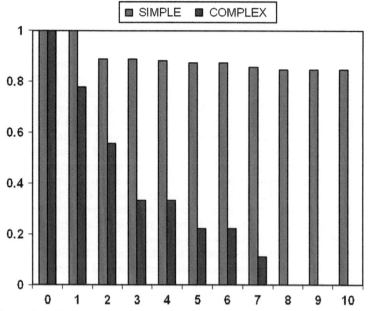

Fig. 2. Sporadic malignant gastrinomas and 10-year survival.

These tumors are small, multiple, and almost always benign. Gastrin is increased in the circulation of these patients as is CgA, similar to what can be observed with chronic potent PPI therapy (see earlier discussion).

Type 2 NETs of the stomach occur because of increased gastrin secretion caused by gastrinoma, most often MEN1. Gastrinomas in MEN1 are frequently multiple and small, and are often treated conservatively. Therefore, gastrin remains high in the circulation on a permanent basis. These patients are treated with PPIs to maintain a neutral pH in the stomach and remove the risk of ulcers and the associated problems. The drive to the ECL cell is increased through the lack of negative feedback in addition to the drive from the gastrinoma. In these patients both gastrin and CgA are increased in the circulation.

Type 3 NETs of the stomach are sporadic, usually solitary, and have a high proliferative index. Gastrin and CgA are not increased in the circulation of these patients although histologic examination confirms neuroendocrine tumor cell characteristics. Prognosis is poor for these patients, and the chance for metastatic spread to the liver is high at the time of diagnosis.

NETs of the Duodenum

Neuroendocrine tumors of the duodenum are rare and usually associated with MEN1. They most often secrete gastrin and, if malignant, may also secrete CgA. Very rarely, tumors of the duodenum may secrete PP or somatostatin or the tachykinins. These tumors may be benign and slow growing.

NETS of the Ileum and Proximal Colon

These tumors are the most common NETs located in the gastrointestinal (GI) tract and are generally small, often solitary, but multifocal in many cases. They secrete serotonin and are commonly referred to as midgut carcinoid (MGC) tumors. As well as serotonin, they secrete CgA and the tachykinins, especially neurokinin A (NKA) and substance P (SP). As the primary tumor may be small, they often go undetected and the patients may present with metastatic disease, which is associated with the typical carcinoid syndrome of flushing and diarrhea, which may be accompanied by palpations, night sweats, broncoconstriction, abdominal pain, pellagra, and over time, right-sided heart disease. These symptoms are a result of the high concentrations of serotonin and the tachykinins that circulate when disease has metastasized to the liver. A significant number of patients, however, present with early disease as the secretory products from the tumor causes local fibrosis and a desmoplastic reaction in the mesentery. This may result in intermittent or acute obstruction even when the primary lesion remains very small. These patients present for surgery without having had circulating biomarkers measured and only postoperative testing is possible. Biomarkers may decrease to within the reference range for CgA, serotonin, and the tachykinins giving a false sense of security of surgical cure when there is no evidence of hepatic spread and local lymph nodes have been dissected with good results. However, it should be noted that surgical cure in these patients is rare and long-term follow-up is essential.

Serotonin has been difficult to measure reliably in serum. Therefore the measurement of its metabolite, 5-hydroxyindole acetic acid (5HIAA) in urine, is the method of choice for assessing serotonin concentration, especially if liver metastasis is suspected, and a 24-hour collection of urine is made. Foods that are high in serotonin and tryptophan must be excluded from the diet for 24 hours preceding and during urine collection. Drugs that affect tryptophan metabolism interfere in the assay also making results unreliable. Some centers measure serum serotonin, but restriction with certain foods and drugs remains important. Recently, more reliable and reproducible serotonin assays have made it possible to monitor midgut carcinoid activity in whole blood.

There are 3 tachykinins that are secreted in humans: neuropeptide K, NKA, and SP. These are produced and secreted in high concentrations by NETs of the ileum and proximal colon.[19,20] As tachykinins circulate in very low concentrations in normal healthy individuals and are increased significantly only in this condition, this offers an excellent alternative method of diagnosis for these tumors.[19] Sensitive assays have been developed for NKA, which is much more stable in blood than SP.

NETs of the Appendix

NETS of the appendix are not uncommon but present at an early stage with appendicitis. With few exceptions, they are benign, are cured surgically, and do not require follow-up (except for those >2 cm in diameter or those sited on the lip of the appendix or invading the mesoappendix). For the small percentage of patients who do require follow-up, then the same range of biomarkers used to diagnose and follow tumors (MGC, urinary 5HIAA, CgA, and NKA) are suggested.

NETs of the Distal Colon and Rectum

It has become apparent that NETs of the distal colon and rectum are much more common than was originally believed. They are small, usually solitary, often benign, and are slow growing. Where a tumor is malignant and small with no metastatic spread to the liver, then again the circulating CgA is not significantly increased. A proportion of these tumors secrete pancreatic polypeptide tyrosine (PPY). PPY assays are commercially available in Europe and in the United States. Some PP assays cross-react with PPY and indicate increased concentrations in these patients. Some NETs of the distal bowel may secrete somatostatin. When a biomarker is found for a particular patient, then this remains a helpful tool to monitor disease.

Pancreastatin is increased when tumors have metastasized to the liver only.[8] It seems to reflect early liver tumor activity.[9]

NETs of Meckel diverticulum are surprisingly common in those individuals who have this particular anatomic abnormality. By the time of diagnosis these tumors have usually metastasized. They secrete CgA and more than half also secrete gastrin.

Secretory products of NETs of the GI tract are shown in **Table 2**.

MEASUREMENT OF CIRCULATING BIOMARKERS FOR NETs

Regulatory peptides have traditionally been measured by radioimmunoassay. This method has offered specificity and sensitivity. With the endeavor to minimize the use of radiochemicals in the laboratory, enzyme-linked immunoassay (ELISA) has been used increasingly and these assays have improved in sensitivity in recent years. There are many commercial assays available for CgA and for the specific peptides biomarkers; many diagnostic laboratories use in-house assays. There are no international standards available and few quality assurance systems, except for insulin and gastrin, thus very strict internal standardization and quality assurance must be in place and only accredited laboratories should be used. There are numerous assays available for the measurement of circulating tumor biomarkers for NETs and many reliable commercial kits.[20,21]

Specimens should be collected a minimum of 6 hours post prandial for the measurement of insulin, gastrin, glucagon, and PP. When CgA and/or gastrin are assayed, it is important that information about PPI therapy is available. Some additional clinical information accompanying the request may be helpful for the diagnostic laboratory as this assists with interpretation of results. In particular, it is important to know if the patient is being treated with somatostatin analogues as this therapy suppresses the secretion of CgA and the regulatory peptides (**Fig. 3**).[22]

Table 2 Secretory products from GI NETs			
Tumor Site	**Syndrome**	**Symptoms**	**Biomarkers**
Gastric (type 1)	None	Upper GI	CgA gastrin
Gastric (type 2)	Usually	Upper GI	CgA gastrin
Gastric (type 3)	None	Upper GI	CgA[b]
Duodenal	Zollinger-Ellison (G)	Epigastric pain (G), peptic ulcer (G), diarrhea (G)	CgA gastrin (>50%), PP (35%), Som (<10%)
Ileal	Carcinoid	Diarrhea, flushing, sweating	CgA, serotonin, NKA, and SP
Appendix	Carcinoid[a]	Diarrhea, flushing, sweating[a]	CgA,[a] serotonin,[a] NKA, and SP[a]
Rectal	None	None	CgA,[a] PYY(10%)
Meckel diverticulum	Zollinger-Ellison (G)	Epigastric pain (G), peptic ulcer (G), diarrhea (G)	CgA, gastrin (>50%)

Abbreviations: G, when gastrin is secreted; Som, somatostatin.
[a] Only if metastatic (appendiceal tumors are rarely metastatic).
[b] CgA may not be secreted if tumor is very poorly differentiated.

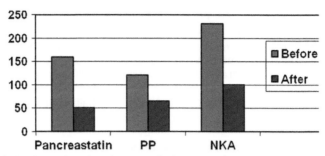

Fig. 3. Circulating biomakers (ng/L) in MGC before and after octreotide (50 μg).

As CgA and regulatory peptides (with the exception of insulin) are processed through the kidney, patients with renal impairment have increased concentrations of these molecules in the circulation. This makes interpretation of results from patients with renal impairment almost impossible.

LABORATORY DIAGNOSIS, MONITORING TREATMENT, AND DETECTING RECURRENT DISEASE

There has been some discussion already regarding the limitations of CgA and regulatory peptides in the diagnosis of NETs. CgA is the only general circulating biomarker for NETs but is poor because of the problems with false-positives. However, it is important to establish a baseline concentration so that treatment and recurrence may be monitored. Gastrin measurement is also inadequate as a sole diagnostic tool for gastrinoma but pretreatment values are required to assess success of treatment or to detect recurrent disease.

There are many advantages to using circulating biomarkers to monitor treatment or detect early recurrence of disease for NETs. The ease of frequent repeat testing, the noninvasive nature of testing and the relatively low cost are persuasive arguments for the ready use of biomarkers for follow-up.

Fig. 4 shows circulating gastrin response to surgery, streptozotocin, and 5-fluorouracil repeated for 3 treatments and then followed by hepatic artery embolization on 2 occasions in a single patient.

The sensitivity of circulating biomarkers to detect changes is most important. As liver metastases may be small and multiple, measurement of circulating biomarkers

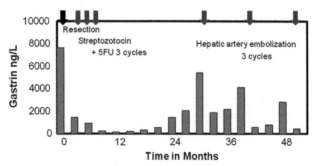

Fig. 4. Gastrin monitoring in a single patient with gastrinoma in a 4-year period during several treatments.

offers earlier indication of advancing disease than radiological techniques. With the increasing options for treatment of liver metastases and disseminated disease, early indication of progression is important.

When disease is inoperable, then circulating biomarkers can indicate stable disease and controlled secretion of active peptides. Retesting at frequent intervals reassures the physician of their choice of treatment. **Fig. 5** illustrates control of MGC achieved for a 3-year period in a single patient with advanced disease who did not respond to somatostatin analogues (SST) alone, but was controlled for more than 7 years when alpha interferon was administered concomitant with SST.

PROGNOSTIC INDICATORS

Because of the variability of tumor progression in NETs from indolent to aggressive and the unpredictable nature of these tumors, prognostic indicators are sought. This makes it possible to avoid over-treating slow-growing tumors and not neglect tumors that will progress rapidly. The window of opportunity for treatment options in aggressive tumors may be narrow.

Several studies have analyzed retrospective data that have resulted in the accumulation of information about several potential prognostic indicators. Age, depth of penetration into the mucosa for tumors in the lumen, metastatic spread, metastatic volume or number of metastases,[23–25] proliferative index,[26] and circulating biomarkers[27] including CgA, pancreastatin and for tumors of the ileum and proximal colon, serotonin concentrations, urinary 5HIAA excretion, and circulating NKA have all been identified as prognostic indicators for tumors of the midgut.[19]

Prognostic indicators identified at surgery or by biopsy relate to a single point in time and it is not possible to assess changing prognosis.[26] The proliferative index (Ki67 or MIB^{-1}) may change with time, and it may not be possible to perform repeat biopsies. Circulating biomarkers, therefore, remain an attractive option for assessing prognosis and for reassessing a potential change in prognosis after treatment. Chromogranin A has been identified as a prognostic indicator with a CgA level greater than 1000 indicating poor prognosis. Pancreastatin has also been used as a prognostic indicator and rapidly increasing pancreastatin measured in an assay that does not cross-react with total molecule CgA has been identified as an indicator of active progressive liver

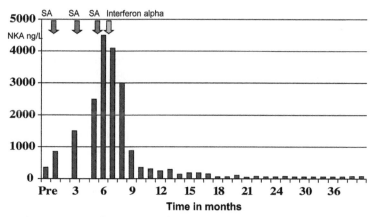

Fig. 5. Circulating NKA used to monitor disease in a single patient with MGC during treatment with somatostatin analogues and alpha interferon.

activity.[8,9] This may be more sensitive than CgA in most patients with extensive metastatic disease. Circulating CgA remains high, more than 30 times more than the reference range.

For the relatively common tumors of the ileum and proximal colon, which frequently have a proliferative index less than 2% yet have a very variable disease progression, both increased urinary 5HIAA and increased NKA have been identified as independent indicators of poor prognosis. NKA is sensitive and specific, and it has also been shown, in a retrospective study, that the most recent NKA estimation is the most accurate indicator of prognosis.[17] Early reports from a prospective study indicated that decreasing NKA in patients with MGC offers longer survival times and it is postulated that circulating NKA not only reflects tumor bulk but also tumor activity.[28]

Circulating biomarkers offer a useful diagnostic tool in conjunction with radiology and tissue pathology for NETs. However, these biomarkers are more reliable when used to monitor disease progression, response to treatment, and for early indication of recurrence after treatment. The increasing use of CgA and pancreastatin as prognostic indicators for NETs in general and the use of NKA for tumors of the midgut in particular offers great potential to assist in decision making for earlier treatment with newly presenting patients and for those with recurring or advancing disease. Although the list of circulating biomarkers that are useful to the clinician who manages these patients is small, they offer readily available and potentially frequent information with noninvasive technology. Additional circulating biomarkers should be sought, particularly in the light of new cellular pathways being explored as therapeutic targets and the potential of personalized treatments becoming a reality.

REFERENCES

1. Ardill JE, Eriksson B. The importance of the measurement of circulating markers in patients with neuroendocrine tumours of the pancreas and gut. Endocr Relat Cancer 2003;10(4):459–62.
2. Öberg K. Biochemical diagnosis of neuroendocrine GEP tumors. Yale J Biol Med 1997;70:501–8.
3. Hutton JC, Davidson HW, Peshavaria M. Proteolytic processing of chromogranin A in purified insulin granules. Formation of a 20 kDa N-terminal fragment (beta-granin) by the concerted action of a Ca^{2+} dependent endopeptidase and carboxypeptidase H (EC 341710). Biochem J 1987;244:457–64.
4. Curry WJ, Johnston CF, Hutton CJ, et al. The tissue distribution of rat chromogranin A-derived peptides: evidence for differential tissue processing from sequence specific antisera. Histochemistry 1991;96:531–8.
5. McGrath-Lindin SJ, Johnston CF, O'Connor DT, et al. Pancreastatin-like immunoreactivity in human carcinoid disease. Regul Pept 1991;33:55–70.
6. Stridsberg M, Öberg K, Li Q, et al. Measurement of chromogranin A, chromogranin B (secretogranin 1) chromogranin C (secretogranin 11) and pancreastatin in plasma and urine from patients with carcinoid tumours and endocrine pancreatic tumours. J Endocrinol 1995;426:361–7.
7. Armstrong L, Ardill JE. Regional laboratory audit to evaluate specificity and sensitivity of chromogranin A and peptide markers in neuroendocrine tumours [abstract]. Regul Pept 2010;164:11. PO12.
8. Stronge RL, Turner GB, Johnston BT, et al. A rapid rise in circulating pancreastatin in response to somatostatin analogue therapy is associated with poor

survival in patients with neuroendocrine tumours. Ann Clin Biochem 2008;45: 560–6.

9. O'Dorisio TM, Krutzik SR, Woltering EA, et al. Development of a highly sensitive and specific carboxy-terminal human pancreastatin assay to monitor neuroendocrine tumor behavior. Pancreas 2010;39(5):611–6.

10. Stridsberg M, Eriksson B, Fellström B, et al. Measurement of Chromogranin B can serve as a complement to chromogranin A. Regul Pept 2007;139:80–3.

11. Duh Q, Hybarger CP, Geist R, et al. Carcinoids associated with multiple endocrine neoplasia syndromes. Am J Surg 1987;154:142–8.

12. Fajans SS, Vinik AI. Insulin-producing islet cell tumors. Endocrinol Metab Clin North Am 1989;18:45–74.

13. Larkin CJ, Ardill JE, Johnston CF, et al. Gastrinomas and the change in their presentation and management in Northern Ireland, UK, from 1970 to 1996. Eur J Gastroenterol Hepatol 1998;10(11):947–52.

14. Dhillo WS, Jayasena CN, Lewis CJ, et al. Plasma gastrin measurement cannot be used to diagnose a gastrinoma in patients on either proton pump inhibitors or histamine type-2 receptor antagonists. Ann Clin Biochem 2006;43:153–5.

15. Frucht H, Howard JM, Slaff JI, et al. Secretin and calcium provocative tests in the Zollinger-Ellison syndrome A prospective study. Ann Intern Med 1989;111(9): 713–22.

16. Dhanvantari S, Seidah NG, Brubaker PL. Role of prohormone convertase in the tissue-specific processing of proglucagon. Mol Endocrinol 1996;10:342–55.

17. Hartmann B, Johnsen AH, Ørskov C, et al. Structure, measurement, and secretion of human glucagon-like peptide-2. Peptides 2000;21(1):73–80.

18. Ardill JE, Fillmore D, Johnston CF, et al. A significant number of spontaneous gastrinomas secrete multiple peptides worsening prognosis. Digestion 1999;60:613 [Abstract].

19. Turner GB, Johnston BT, McCance DR, et al. Circulating markers of prognosis and response to treatment with midgut carcinoid tumours. Gut 2006;55: 1586–91.

20. Ardill JE. Circulating markers for endocrine tumours of the gastroenteropancreatic tract. Ann Clin Biochem 2008;45(6):539–59 [Review].

21. Mamikunian G, Vinik AI, O'Dorisio TM, et al. Neuroendocrine tumors a comprehensive guide to diagnosis and management. Available at: www.interscineceinstitute. com. Accessed September 1, 2010.

22. Shi W, Buchanan KD, Johnston CF, et al. The octreotide suppression test and [111In-DTPA-D-Phe1]-octreotide scintigraphy in neuroendocrine tumours correlate with responsiveness to somatostatin analogue treatment. Clin Endocrinol (Oxf) 1998;48(3):303–9.

23. Ahmed A, Turner G, King B, et al. Midgut neuroendocrine tumours with liver metastases: results of the UKINETS study. Endocr Relat Cancer 2009;16(3): 885–94.

24. Shebani KO, Souba WW, Finkelstein DM, et al. Prognosis and survival in patients with gastrointestinal tract carcinoid tumors. Ann Surg 1999;229(6):815–21 [discussion: 822–3].

25. Burke AP, Thomas RM, Elsayed AM, et al. Carcinoids of the jejunum and ileum: an immunohistochemical and clinicopathologic study of 167 cases. Cancer 1997; 79(6):1086–93.

26. Chaudhry A, Öberg K, Wilander E. A study of biological behavior based on the expression of a proliferating antigen in neuroendocrine tumors of the digestive system. Tumour Biol 1992;13(1–2):27–35.

27. Janson ET, Holmberg L, Stridsberg M, et al. Carcinoid tumors: analysis of prognostic factors and survival in 301 patients from a referral center. Ann Oncol 1997; 8(7):685–90.
28. Ardill JE, Armstrong L, McCance DR, et al. Neurokinin A is a sensitive marker and excellent prognostic indicator for serotonin secreting tumours of the ileum and colon. Regul Pept 2010;164:7. OC04.

Glucagonlike Peptide-1 Receptor: An Example of Translational Research in Insulinomas: A Review

Emanuel Christ, MD, PhD[a], Damian Wild, MD[b,c],
Jean Claude Reubi, MD[d,*]

KEYWORDS

• Glucagonlike peptide-1 • Glucagonlike petide-1 receptor
• Insulinoma • ^{111}In-DOTA/DPTA-exendin-4

Glucagonlike peptide 1 (GLP-1) is considered to be one of the most important glucose-dependent insulin secretagogues released mainly from the small intestine in response to nutrient intake.[1] The corresponding GLP-1 receptor (GLP-1R) has been identified.[2] It is a member of the class 2 G protein–coupled receptor family[1,3] and is mainly expressed in the pancreatic islet cells, the intestine, lung, kidney, breast, and the brainstem.[4] GLP-1 plays not only an important role in enhancing glucose-dependent insulin biosynthesis and secretion but also in reducing glucagon secretion, decreasing beta cell apoptosis, increasing differentiation of beta cell precursor cells, decreasing gastric emptying, and appetite at the hypothalamic level.[5] It is, therefore, an ideal therapeutic concept for patients with type 2 diabetes that tackles the main pathophysiological mechanism of the disease.[5]

It is a general rule that peptides are extremely rapidly degraded in the human body because of breakdown by potent peptidases.[6] Accordingly, the half-life of GLP-1 is less than 2 minutes[6] because of the efficient degradation by dipeptidyl-peptidase-4

[a] Division of Endocrinology, Diabetology, and Clinical Nutrition, University Hospital of Berne Inselspital, Freiburgstrasse 15, CH 3010 Berne, Switzerland
[b] Department of Nuclear Medicine, University Hospital Freiburg, Hugstetterstrasse 50, D 79106 Freiburg, Germany
[c] Institute of Nuclear Medicine, University College London, 235 Euston Road, London NW1 2BU, UK
[d] Division of Cell Biology and Experimental Cancer Research, Institute of Pathology, University of Berne, PO Box 62, Murtenstrasse 31, CH 3010 Berne, Switzerland
* Corresponding author.
E-mail address: reubi@pathology.unibe.ch

Endocrinol Metab Clin N Am 39 (2010) 791–800
doi:10.1016/j.ecl.2010.09.003
0889-8529/10/$ – see front matter © 2010 Elsevier Inc. All rights reserved.

(DPP-4). Exendin-4 is a naturally occurring peptide identified in the saliva of the Gila monster (*Heloderma suspectum*). Exendin-4 is a larger molecule (39 amino acids instead of 30) than human GLP-1 and shares 53% homology with the human GLP-1.[1] The molecular structure makes it resistant to degradation by DPP-4.[1] A synthetic version of exendin-4 is approved by the Food and Drug Administration (FDA) and the European Medicines Agency (EMEA) for the treatment of type 2 diabetes.[5]

G protein–coupled peptide hormone receptors play an increasing role in cancer medicine.[7] The underlying pathophysiological mechanism is primarily an overexpression of a specific peptide receptor on tumor cells that allows diagnostic (receptor-targeted scintigraphic tumor imaging) and therapeutic procedures using radiolabeled peptide analogs.[7] Historically, the somatostatin receptors were the first receptors identified for these purposes.[7] These receptors are homogeneously expressed in high density on gastroenteropancreatic neuroendocrine tumors.[7] Somatostatin receptor scintigraphy using the somatostatin analog—octreotide (OctreoScan)—became an integral part of the routine diagnostic procedures in patients with neuroendocrine tumors. In addition, results from clinical studies performing somatostatin receptor-mediated radionuclide therapy are encouraging.[8]

A new potentially promising candidate for in vivo targeting is the GLP-1R.[9] This review summarizes the current knowledge of GLP-1R targeting in vitro and in animal models, and provides preliminary data of diagnostic imaging in humans.

GLP-1R KNOCK OUT AND GLP-1R OVEREXPRESSION

Only a single GLP-1R has been identified so far that is structurally identical in all tissues.[2] Upon agonist binding of GLP-1 or exendin-4 to GLP-1R, stimulation of adenylate cyclase and phospholipase C with subsequent activation of PKA and PKC, respectively, is triggered, which results in the insulinotropic effects described previously.[2]

Mice with a targeted disruption of the GLP-1R gene have been used to understand the biologic importance of GLP-1.[10] GLP-1R$^{-/-}$ mice exhibit relatively modest perturbation of glucose homeostasis: they have mild fasting hyperglycemia and glucose intolerance after an oral glucose challenge in association with a reduction in glucose-stimulated insulin secretion.[10] However, although GLP-1 is a potent inhibitor of short-term food intake, GLP-1R$^{-/-}$ mice show normal body weight and food intake suggesting alternative pathways for the regulation of nutritional regime.[10]

Conversely, a model of GLP-1R overexpression has been reported in an insulinoma cell line.[11] In GLP-R transfected cells, glucose-mediated insulin release was increased compared with the control cells, in parallel with an increase in the intracellular second messenger of the GLP-1R (cAMP).[11]

GLP-1R IN VARIOUS TISSUES

In humans and rodents, GLP-1R is expressed in various tissues including the α, β, and δ cells of the islets of Langerhans, lung, stomach, heart, intestine, kidney, and the brainstem, hypothalamus, and pituitary.[4,12] In humans, the highest GLP-1R expression is observed in neurohypophysis, followed by the duodenum (Brunner's gland) and the pancreatic islets.[12] With the exception of Brunner's gland of the duodenum, the different tissues in the proximity of the pancreas islets (ie, pancreas acini, intestine, and kidney) exhibit only about 50% of the GLP-1R density compared with the islets.[12] It appears that there are some important species differences in GLP-1R expression: autoradiography experiments in rats and mice indicate that GLP-1R density is several fold higher in the lungs of rodents compared with the corresponding human tissue.[12]

Similarly, GLP-1R density in the thyroid gland is higher in rodents than in humans.[12] Interestingly, thyroid C-cell hyperplasia and medullary carcinoma have been demonstrated in rodents following therapy with GLP-1 analogs, whereas in studies with GLP-1 analogs in humans there is so far no evidence for such complications. It can be speculated whether the species differences in GLP-1R density expression contribute to these controversial findings.

GLP-1R IN TUMORS

Recently, GLP-1R incidence and density has been determined in vitro in a broad spectrum of human tumors[9,12] using the autoradiography technique (**Fig. 1**). The most striking incidence and density of GLP-1R was found in insulinomas, an usually benign insulin-secreting neuroendocrine tumor of the pancreas (incidence: 93%, mean density 8100 degradation per minutes per mg [dpm/mg] tissue [**Fig. 2**]).[9] Also, gastrinomas express GLP-1R in most cases, however, with a lower density.[9]

In endocrine tumors, such as phaeochromocytomas, GLP-1R has been detected in 60% with a relatively high density (nearly 4000 dpm/mg tissue); the incidence in paraganglioma and medullary thyroid carcinomas is lower (28%) with a mean density of about 1350 dpm/mg tissue.[12] It is noteworthy that in pituitary adenomas and adrenal cortical adenoma, GLP-1R has not been identified.[12]

GLP-1R is absent in epithelial tumors such as breast, colorectal, gastric, pancreatic, hepatocellular, and cholangiocellular as well as in lung carcinomas (non–small and

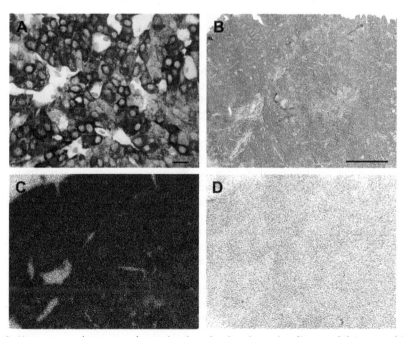

Fig. 1. Hormone and receptor determinations in vitro in an insulinoma. (*A*) Immunohistochemistry for insulin showing strongly labeled tumor cells. Bar = 0.01 mm. (*B*) Hematoxylin-eosin–stained tumor tissue used for autoradiography. Bar = 1 mm. (*C*) Autoradiogram showing total binding of ^{125}I-GLP-1(7-36) amide. Whole tumor is strongly positive. (*D*) Autoradiogram showing nonspecific binding of ^{125}I-GLP-1(7-36) amide in the presence of 100 NM GLP1(7-36) amide.

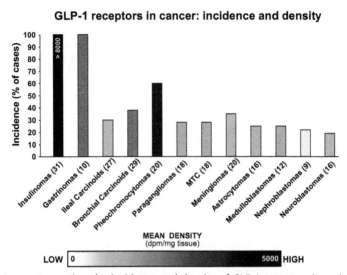

Fig. 2. Histogram reporting the incidence and density of GLP-1 receptors in various human cancers. Darkness of the bars represents receptor density from 0 to 5000 dpm/mg tissue. Mean density in insulinomas is more than 8000 dpm/mg. Number of tested cases are in parentheses.

small cell carcinoma.[12] Ovarian and prostate carcinomas have a low incidence of GLP-1R (5%–15%).[12] Non-Hodgkin lymphomas do not exhibit GLP-1Rs, whereas embryonic tumors (medullobastoma, nephroblastoma, and neuroblastoma) show GLP-1R in 15% to 25% of the tumors with a mean GLP-1R density of about 400 to 1200 dpm/mg.[12] Tumors of the nervous system, such as meningioma and astrocytoma, demonstrate an incidence of GLP-1R between 25% and 35%, whereas in glioblastoma and ependymoma the incidence is somehow lower (9%–16%).[12] Schwannomas are devoid of GLP-1R.[12]

Based on the following considerations, the particular high incidence and density of GLP-1R on insulinomas are of particular clinical interest: (1) in contrast to the gastro-enteropancreatic neuroendocrine tumors, insulinomas express less frequently somatostatin receptors. OctreoScan, therefore, is not a reliable tool to detect these lesions.[13] (2) The exact intraoperative localization of the insulinoma is critical to minimize surgical intervention[14]; however, benign insulinoma are usually small (10–20 mm) and difficult to localize using conventional radiological procedures (endosonography, MR- and CT-imaging technique).[15] The amine precursor fluorine-18-L-dihydroxyphe-nylalanine ([18F]DOPA) shows, for the moment, controversial results with sensitivities ranging from 17% up to 90%.[16,17] Although selective arterial stimulated and venous sampling is a reliable tool in an experienced institution,[18] it is an invasive procedure with the associated risks. Furthermore, this procedure identifies only the region of the pancreas, depending on the vasculature, where the insulinoma should be located and not always the tumor itself.[18]

Based on the previously mentioned findings, it appears appropriate to further explore the possibility of targeting human conditions with endogenous hyperinsuline-mic hypoglycemia. A prerequisite for that is to evaluate first the targeting of GLP-1R in animal models of insulinomas. This requires adequate radioligands as tools and an adequate animal tumor model (see later in this article).

GLP-1R ANALOGS

In general, radiopeptides are small, usually devoid of side effects, and characterized by their fast diffusion, lack of immunogenicity, and fast blood clearance.[7] In addition, radiolabeling is easily feasible, preferably after attaching a chelator to the peptide.[19] Initially, GLP-1R targeting was performed with ^{125}I labeled GLP-1 and the GLP-1 analog exendin-3.[20] However, the low peptide stability of GLP-1 and the low efficiency of radio iodination of exendin-3 limit their clinical use.[20] Further testing resulted in the development of the GLP-1R analog exendin-4 that shares 53% homology with GLP-1, but is considerably more stable than GLP-1.[21] Exendin-4 has been coupled via the Lys side chain to a chelator (DOTA [tetraazacyclododecantetraacetic acid] or DTPA [diethylenetriaminepentacetic acid]) using a spacer (Ahx [aminohexanoic acid][21]; **Fig. 3**). This whole molecule has been successfully labeled with ^{111}In and in vitro and in vivo characterization (GLP-1R binding, internalization kinetics, biodistribution) of this radiopeptide has been obtained in an animal insulinoma tumor model.[21,22] Recently, 2 studies have been published that describe two ^{68}Ga-labeled GLP-1 receptor agonists (^{68}Ga-DOTA-exendin-4 and ^{68}Ga-DOTA-exendin-3) for positron emission tomography (PET)/CT imaging and one ^{99m}Tc-labeled GLP-1 receptor agonist (^{99m}Tc-HYNIC-exendin-4) for single-photon emission computed tomography (SPECT)/CT imaging.[23,24]

GLP-1R TARGETING IN ANIMAL MODELS

Initially, GLP-1R targeting was performed in a rat insulinoma animal model (NEDH rats) and in rat insulinoma cell line (RINm5F) using ^{125}I-labeled GLP-1 and exendin-3, an analog of GLP-1.[20] Specific uptake was detected in the cell and animal model, further substantiating the principle of proof for GLP-1R targeting in insulinoma.[20] However, because of the short half-life of GLP-1 and difficulties in labeling exendin-3, this radiopeptide was abandoned for clinical use.[20]

Later, a mouse model was used, the Rip1tag2 transgenic mice. They develop tumors of the pancreatic beta cells in a reproducible multistage tumor progression pathway[25] and represent, therefore, an ideal model to study GLP-1R targeting in vivo and in vitro. Using GLP-1R imaging with multipinhole SPECT/MRI and SPECT/CT, GLP-1R imaging was performed in these animals following administration of ^{111}In-DTPA-exendin-4.[21] In parallel, autoradiography of the tumors was performed

Scheme of the radiopeptide for GLP-1 targeting

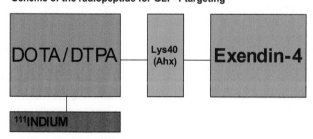

[Lys40(Ahx-DOTA/DTPA-111In)NH2]exendin-4

Fig. 3. Exendin-4 is coupled via the Lys side chain to a chelator (DOTA [tetraazacyclododecantetraacetic acid] or DTPA [diethylenetriaminepentacetic acid]) using a spacer (Ahx [aminohexanoic acid]). This whole molecule is successfully labeled with [111]Indium as a tracer.

and, finally, using tumor cells derived from this animal model, internalization, cellular retention, biodistribution, and pharmacokinetics of ^{111}In-DTPA-exendin-4 were studied.[21]

This preclinical study showed the following main findings: (1) the GLP-1R density in the tumors was extremely high resulting in a remarkably high uptake of ^{111}In-DTPA-exendin-4 (287% ± 62% IA/g tissue) already 4 hours after injection; (2) excellent tumor visualization (minimal tumor size of 1–3 mm) by pinhole SPECT/MRI and PECT/CT was demonstrated; (3) the tumor-to-background ratio was very high (between 13.6 and 299.0), corroborating the high potential of this radiopetide to specifically localize GLP-1R-positive lesions within the pancreas; And (4) in vitro studies in the cell-derived model demonstrated a specific internalization of ^{111}In-DTPA-exendin-4 and biochemical investigations confirm high metabolic stability in serum and tumor cells.

There are preliminary data on GLP-1R-targeted therapy in the same Rip1Tag2 mouse model. Mice were injected with different doses of ^{111}In-DTPA-exendin-4 (1.1, 5.6, and 28.0 MBq) and humanely killed 7 days after injection. Most impressively, a single injection led to a reduction in tumor volume of up to 94% in a dose-dependent manner without significant acute organ toxicity. Histologic examination revealed that the decrease in tumor mass was mainly because of an increase in tumor cell apoptosis and decreased proliferation.[22]

GLP-1R TARGETING IN HUMANS

Based on the encouraging preclinical results, ^{111}In-DOTA-exendin-4 was prospectively administered to 6 patients.[26] All of them presented with neuroglycopenic symptoms lasting for 4 to 26 months. Biochemical evaluation during a fasting test revealed endogenous hyperinsulinemic hypoglycemia in all patients. Conventional imaging (CT or MRI) reliably detected the insulinoma in only 2 patients, whereas endosonography identified a possible lesion in 4 patients, in keeping with data in the literature.[27] In 3 patients, selective arterial stimulation and venous sampling was performed with correct localization in all 3 patients.[26] Remarkably, GLP1-R scintigraphy correctly detected the insulinoma in all 6 consecutive patients.[26] Four patients underwent an enucleation of the insulinoma. In 2 patients, a Whipple procedure had to be performed because of the localization of the insulinoma. In all patients, benign insulinoma was confirmed by histology. In vitro autoradiography of GLP-1R showed a density of GLP-1R in the range as previously described (between 2600 and >10,000 dpm/mg tissue)[9]; whereas somatostatin receptor status revealed low levels of somatostatin-1 receptor subtype in 2 patients only.[26] Importantly, within a time frame of 2 to 14 days after injection of ^{111}In-DOTA-exendin-4, intraoperative use of a gamma probe was highly beneficial for the in situ localization in all patients resulting in a successful enucleation where possible (**Fig. 4**).[26]

Interestingly, in 1 of the 6 patients GLP-1R scintigraphy revealed an increased extrapancreatic uptake in the mesentery supplied by the anterior mesentery artery. Selective arterial stimulation and venous sampling correctly indicated the vascular territory, but because this patient had an ectopic insulinoma, the results of the invasive investigation without GLP-1R imaging would have been misleading for the surgical strategy.[28]

Fortunately, background uptake over the whole body was low with the exception of the kidneys, which were strongly labeled owing to renal excretion of the radioligand. In 2 patients, demarcation between tumors (maximal diameter of 9–11 mm) and kidneys was possible only after late scans, indicating an improved tumor-to-kidney ratio with time in keeping with the fact that the effective half-life of ^{111}In-DOTA-exendin-4 was

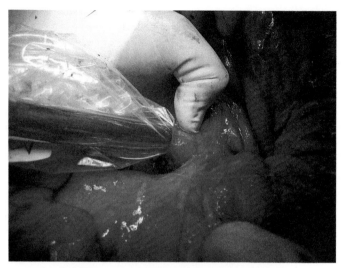

Fig. 4. Intraoperative detection of insulinoma using a gamma probe.

longer in the tumor (38–64 hours) than in the kidneys (31.2–31.8 hours).[26] This suggests that patients with negative early scans should have additional imaging 3 to 7 days after the injection.

In humans, DOTA was initially administered, but later replaced by DTPA because of the 4 times higher specific activity of ^{111}In-DTPA-exendin-4 compared with ^{111}In-DOTA-exendin-4 (**Fig. 5**).[29] A higher specific activity permits reduction of the amount of peptide (exendin-4), thereby decreasing the occurrence of possible side effects. In addition, radiolabeling of DTPA-exendin-4 can be performed at room temperature, whereas labeling of DOTA-exendin-4 has to be done at high temperature (95°C).[21] **Fig. 5** shows ^{111}In-DTPA-exendin-4 whole-body planar images and a ^{111}In-DTPA-exendin-4 SPECT/CT scan from a patient with a histology-proven benign insulinoma in the head of pancreas. Preliminary data of an ongoing study using ^{111}In-DPTA-exendin-4 confirm the previous findings.[30]

About 90% of insulinomas are benign and only 10% of patients present with malignant disease, usually characterized by liver metastasis.[13] Anecdotal evidence suggests that malignant insulinomas more often exhibit sst_2 receptors than benign and can, therefore, be visualized by OctreoScan.[13] Preliminary data with 10 patients with malignant insulinoma indicate that sst_2 receptors are expressed in 7 patients, whereas GLP-1R was present in 4 patients and both receptors in only 1 patient.[30] Importantly, 1 of the 2 imaging methods appears always to be positive in a malignant type of insulinoma.[30]

SIDE EFFECTS AND LIMITATIONS

In humans, the injection of ^{111}In-DOTA-exendin-4 and ^{111}In-DPTA-exendin-4 was well tolerated. Because of the small amount of exendin-4, the decrease in plasma glucose concentrations was only 1.4 ± 0.7 mmol/L after 40 minutes.[26] By regularly monitoring glucose levels, no severe hypoglycemic episode occurred. One patient experienced a short episode of vomiting; otherwise, no further side effects were observed.[26]

In 2 patients, there was focal ^{111}In-DOTA-exendin-4 uptake in the proximal duodenum. As previously mentioned, this may be related to the presence of

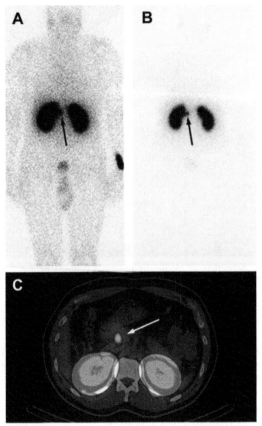

Fig. 5. ^{111}In-DTPA-exendin-4 whole-body planar images (*A, B*) and ^{111}In-DTPA-exendin-4 SPECT/CT scan (*C*) from a patient with a histology-proven benign insulinoma. Whole-body scans were performed at 4 hours (*A*) and 120 hours (*B*) after injection, whereas the SPECT/CT scan was done 4 hours after injection of 98 MBq (10 μg) ^{111}In-DTPA-exendin-4. The arrow indicates the location of the insulinoma in the head of pancreas (*A–C*). The longest residence time of ^{111}In-DTPA-exendin-4 was observed in the tumor (*arrow*) and kidneys (*B*).

Brunner's glands of the duodenum, which are known to contain GLP-1Rs in a significant density.[12] Brunner's glands may become hyperplastic,[31] as observed in particular in patients with chronic pancreatitis.[32] Such hyperplastic glands may possibly be detected by GLP-1R imaging.

A differential diagnosis of endogenous hyperinsulinemic hypoglycemia includes nesidioblastosis, defined as a diffuse hyperplasia of beta-cells occurring usually in children.[33] Recent evidence suggests that this pathology can also be demonstrated in adults, in particular after bypass-surgery for morbid obesity.[34] Presently, there is no in vitro or in vivo evidence suggesting that GLP-1R is expressed in sufficient density to allow detection by scintigraphy. However, ^{18}F-DOPA-PET has successfully been used to detect nesidioblastosis and benign insulinoma.[16] However, tumor:background ratios are higher for ^{111}In-DOTA-exendin-4 SPECT than for ^{18}F-DOPA-PET (3.3 vs 1.4), suggesting an increased sensitivity of targeting GLP-1Rs, at least in benign insulinomas.[16,26]

SUMMARY AND CONCLUSION

GLP-1R plays an increasingly important role in endocrine gastrointestinal tumor management. Targeting GLP-1R by ^{111}In-DOTA-exendin-4 or ^{111}In-DPTA-exendin-4 offers a new approach that permits the successful localization of small insulinomas pre- and intraoperatively. Because virtually all benign insulinomas express GLP-1Rs, it is likely that this approach will affect the algorithm of pre- and intraoperative localization of suspected insulinoma. If the high sensitivity and specificity are confirmed in the future, it is likely that this new technique will replace the invasive localization by selective arterial stimulation and venous sampling.

REFERENCES

1. Nauck MA. Unraveling the science of incretin biology. Eur J Intern Med 2009; 20(Suppl 2):S303–8.
2. Thorens B, Porret A, Buhler L, et al. Cloning and functional expression of the human islet GLP-1 receptor. Demonstration that exendin-4 is an agonist and exendin-(9-39) an antagonist of the receptor. Diabetes 1993;42(11):1678–82.
3. Gros L, Thorens B, Bataille D, et al. Glucagon-like peptide-1-(7-36) amide, oxyntomodulin, and glucagon interact with a common receptor in a somato-statin-secreting cell line. Endocrinology 1993;133(2):631–8.
4. Wei Y, Mojsov S. Tissue-specific expression of the human receptor for glucagon-like peptide-I: brain, heart and pancreatic forms have the same deduced amino acid sequences. FEBS Lett 1995;358(3):219–24.
5. Nauck MA, Vilsboll T, Gallwitz B, et al. Incretin-based therapies: viewpoints on the way to consensus. Diabetes Care 2009;32(Suppl 2):S223–31.
6. Baggio LL, Drucker DJ. Biology of incretins: GLP-1 and GIP. Gastroenterology 2007;132(6):2131–57.
7. Reubi JC. Peptide receptors as molecular targets for cancer diagnosis and therapy. Endocr Rev 2003;24(4):389–427.
8. Kwekkeboom DJ, de Herder WW, Kam BL, et al. Treatment with the radiolabeled somatostatin analog [177 Lu-DOTA 0, Tyr3]octreotate: toxicity, efficacy, and survival. J Clin Oncol 2008;26(13):2124–30.
9. Reubi JC, Waser B. Concomitant expression of several peptide receptors in neuroendocrine tumors as molecular basis for in vivo multireceptor tumor target-ing. Eur J Nucl Med 2003;30(5):781–93.
10. Hansotia T, Drucker DJ. GIP and GLP-1 as incretin hormones: lessons from single and double incretin receptor knockout mice. Regul Pept 2005;128(2):125–34.
11. Montrose-Rafizadeh C, Wang Y, Janczewski AM, et al. Overexpression of glucagon-like peptide-1 receptor in an insulin-secreting cell line enhances glucose responsiveness. Mol Cell Endocrinol 1997;130(1–2):109–17.
12. Korner M, Stockli M, Waser B, et al. GLP-1 receptor expression in human tumors and human normal tissues: potential for in vivo targeting. J Nucl Med 2007;48(5):736–43.
13. Plockinger U, Rindi G, Arnold R, et al. Guidelines for the diagnosis and treatment of neuroendocrine gastrointestinal tumours. Neuroendocrinology 2004;80(6):394–424.
14. Rostambeigi N, Thompson GB. What should be done in an operating room when an insulinoma cannot be found? Clin Endocrinol (Oxf) 2009;70(4):512–5.
15. Chatziioannou A, Kehagias D, Mourikis D, et al. Imaging and localization of pancreatic insulinomas. Clin Imaging 2001;25(4):275–83.

16. Kauhanen S, Seppanen M, Minn H, et al. Fluorine-18-L-dihydroxyphenylalanine (18F-DOPA) positron emission tomography as a tool to localize an insulinoma or beta-cell hyperplasia in adult patients. J Clin Endocrinol Metab 2007;92(4): 1237–44.

17. Tessonnier L, Sebag F, Ghander C, et al. Limited value of 18F-F-DOPA PET to localize pancreatic insulin-secreting tumors in adults with hyperinsulinemic hypoglycemia. J Clin Endocrinol Metab 2010;95(1):303–7.

18. Wiesli P, Brandle M, Schmid C, et al. Selective arterial calcium stimulation and hepatic venous sampling in the evaluation of hyperinsulinemic hypoglycemia: potential and limitations. J Vasc Interv Radiol 2004;15(11):1251–6.

19. Reubi JC, Maecke HR. Peptide-based probes for cancer imaging. J Nucl Med 2008;49(11):1735–8.

20. Gotthardt M, Fischer M, Naeher I, et al. Use of the incretin hormone glucagon-like peptide-1 (GLP-1) for the detection of insulinomas: initial experimental results. Eur J Nucl Med Mol Imaging 2002;29(5):597–606.

21. Wild D, Behe M, Wicki A, et al. [Lys40(Ahx-DTPA-111In)NH2]Exendin-4, a very promising ligand for glucagon-like peptide-1 (GLP-1) receptor targeting. J Nucl Med 2006;47(12):2025–33.

22. Wicki A, Wild D, Storch D, et al. [Lys40(Ahx-DTPA-111In)NH2]-Exendin-4 is a highly efficient radiotherapeutic for glucagon-like peptide-1 receptor-targeted therapy for insulinoma. Clin Cancer Res 2007;13(12):3696–705.

23. Brom M, Oyen WJ, Joosten L, et al. (68)Ga-labelled exendin-3, a new agent for the detection of insulinomas with PET. Eur J Nucl Med Mol Imaging 2010;37(7):1345–55.

24. Wild D, Wicki A, Mansi R, et al. Exendin-4-based radiopharmaceuticals for glucagon-like peptide-1 (GLP-1) receptor PET/CT and SPECT/CT imaging. J Nucl Med 2010;51(7):1059–67.

25. Hanahan D. Heritable formation of pancreatic beta-cell tumours in transgenic mice expressing recombinant insulin/simian virus 40 oncogenes. Nature 1985; 315(6015):115–22.

26. Christ E, Wild D, Forrer F, et al. Glucagon-like peptide-1 receptor imaging for localization of insulinomas. J Clin Endocrinol Metab 2009;94(11):4398–405.

27. McAuley G, Delaney H, Colville J, et al. Multimodality preoperative imaging of pancreatic insulinomas. Clin Radiol 2005;60(10):1039–50.

28. Wild D, Mäcke H, Christ E, et al. Glucagon-like peptide 1-receptor scans to localize occult insulinomas. N Engl J Med 2008;359(7):766–8.

29. Wild D, Christ E, Forrer F, et al. 111In-DTPA-exendin-4 SPECT/CT scans localize hardly detectable insulinomas. J Nucl Med 2009;50(Suppl 2):1937.

30. Christ E, Wild D, Caplin M, et al. Glucagon-like peptide-1 compared with somato-statin receptor2 targeting in malignant insulinoma [abstract]. Endocrine Soc Meeting 2010, in press.

31. Levine JA, Burgart LJ, Batts KP, et al. Brunner's gland hamartomas: clinical presentation and pathological features of 27 cases. Am J Gastroenterol 1995; 90(2):290–4.

32. Stolte M, Schwabe H, Prestele H. Relationship between diseases of the pancreas and hyperplasia of Brunner's glands. Virchows Arch A Pathol Anat Histol 1981; 394(1–2):75–87.

33. Yakovac WC, Baker L, Hummeler K. Beta cell nesidioblastosis in idiopathic hypoglycemia of infancy. J Pediatr 1971;79(2):226–31.

34. Service GJ, Thompson GB, Service FJ, et al. Hyperinsulinemic hypoglycemia with nesidioblastosis after gastric-bypass surgery. N Engl J Med 2005;353(3): 249–54.

Signaling Mechanisms in Neuroendocrine Tumors as Targets for Therapy

Barbara Zarebczan, MD, Herbert Chen, MD*

KEYWORDS

- Neuroendocrine tumor • Carcinoid • Medullary thyroid cancer
- Signaling pathways

Neuroendocrine tumors (NETs) are rare, with an incidence of 2 to 5 per 100,000 people.[1] These tumors secrete hormones such as 5-hydroxytryptamine (5-HT) (serotonin), chromogranin A (CgA), neuron-specific enolase (NSE), and synaptophysin. These hormones can cause debilitating symptoms of carcinoid syndrome in patients with neuroendocrine malignancies, such as flushing, diarrhea, heart palpitations, and congestive heart failure. NETs also frequently metastasize to the liver long before they are diagnosed, making curative resection unlikely. Traditional methods of cancer treatment, such as chemotherapy, have not been successful in the treatment of NETs. Therefore, it is imperative that new therapies targeting the signaling pathways involved in NETs are developed.

Many of the signaling pathways, which are now known to play an important role in the development and progression of NETs, were initially discovered and studied in other cancers. The phosphatidylinositol 3-kinase (PI3K)-Akt pathway has been well characterized in ovarian cancer, breast cancer, melanoma, and colon cancer.[2,3] Inhibition of this pathway suppresses the growth of both small cell lung cancers and gastrointestinal carcinoids.[4,5] Similarly, Notch1 was first studied as an oncogene in pancreatic cancer, colon cancer, non–small cell lung cancer, and various lymphomas.[6–8] It was then discovered that Notch1 plays the role of tumor suppressor in small cell lung cancer, pancreatic carcinoids, and medullary thyroid cancer.[9–11] The Ras/Raf/mitogen-activated protein kinase (MEK)/extracellular signal–regulated kinase (ERK) pathway has also been reported to play an oncogenic role in colon cancer, lung cancer, and

This work was supported by the American College of Surgeons Research Fellowship Award (B.Z.) and National Institutes of Health T32 Training Grant (B.Z.).
Endocrine Surgery Research Laboratories, Department of Surgery, University of Wisconsin Carbone Cancer Center, 3028 Wisconsin Institutes for Medical Research, 1111 Highland Avenue, Madison, WI 53705, USA
* Corresponding author. H4/722 Clinical Science Center, 600 Highland Avenue, Madison, WI 53792.
E-mail address: chen@surgery.wisc.edu

Endocrinol Metab Clin N Am 39 (2010) 801–810
doi:10.1016/j.ecl.2010.08.002
0889-8529/10/$ – see front matter © 2010 Elsevier Inc. All rights reserved.

melanoma but a tumor suppressive role in NETs, including small cell lung cancers, medullary thyroid cancer, and carcinoid tumors.[12] Finally, the RET pathway, although shown to have a role in papillary thyroid cancer, breast cancer, and melanoma, has been most extensively studied in medullary thyroid cancer.[13–15]

THE PI3K-AKT PATHWAY

The PI3K-Akt pathway plays a role in cell proliferation, survival, and motility.[2] PI3Ks are heterodimer lipid kinases composed of 2 subunits, p85 and p110, which are activated by receptor tyrosine kinases (**Fig. 1**). Once activated, PI3Ks catalyze the conversion of phosphatidylinositol 4,5-bisphosphate (PIP$_2$) to phosphatidylinositol 3,4,5-triphosphate (PIP$_3$), which can be converted back into PIP$_2$ by phosphatase and tensin homolog (PTEN), a 3' phosphatase. PIP$_3$ in turn plays a role in the activation of the

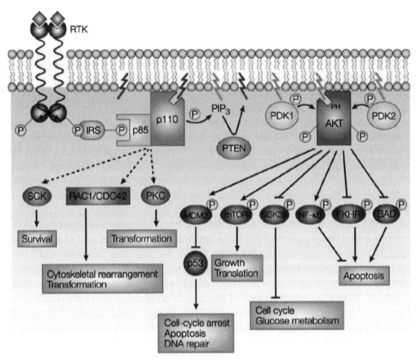

Fig. 1. The PI3K-Akt pathway becomes activated via stimulation of receptor tyrosine kinases (RTKs) and the assembly of receptor-PI3K complexes. The complex then catalyzes the conversion of PIP$_2$ to PIP$_3$. PIP$_3$ then helps to activate Akt. The activated Akt then mediates the activation and inhibition of several targets, includingglycogen synthase kinase-3β (GSK-3β), mammalian target of rapamycin (mTOR), and nuclear factor κB (NF-κB), resulting in cellular growth, metabolism, and survival. BAD, Bcl-2-associated death promoter; CDC42, cell division control protein 42; FKHR, forkhead in human rhabdomyosarcoma; IRS, insulin receptor substrate; MDM2, murine double minute-2 protein; P, phosphate; PDK, phosphoinositide-dependent kinase; PH, pleckstrin homology domain; PIP$_2$, phosphatidylinositol 4,5-bisphosphate; PIP$_3$, phosphatidylinositol 3,4,5-triphosphate; PKC, protein kinase C; PTEN, phosphatase and tensin homolog; RAC1, Ras-related C3 botulinum toxin substrate 1; SGK, serum and glucocorticoid-induced protein kinase. (*From* Vivanco I, Sawyers C. The phosphatidylinositol 3-kinase AKT pathway in human cancer. Nat Rev Cancer 2002;2(7):495; Macmillan Publishers Ltd; with permission.)

serine/threonine protein kinase Akt. There are 3 isoforms of Akt, but Akt1 is the isoform mainly studied in cancers. Akt2 is found in tissues responding to insulin and Akt3 is found in the brain.[16] Akt activates and inhibits several target genes such as nuclear factor κB, mammalian target of rapamycin (mTOR), and glycogen synthase kinase-3β (GSK-3β), all of which have been implicated in various cancers.

Many patients with these cancers have been found to have either mutations in the p85 or p110 subunit or a loss-of-function mutation in PTEN, which then leads to unregulated activation of Akt.[2,3] Pulmonary carcinoid cells have been shown to contain high levels of phosphorylated Akt at baseline, and when treated with an Akt-specific small interfering RNA, these cells demonstrated decreased growth.[16] The same findings were seen in gastrointestinal carcinoid cells, and these tumors have been shown to have a loss of PTEN function.[5,17,18] Similarly, upregulation of the PI3K-Akt pathway via a loss of PTEN function has been implicated in the development of up to 15% of small cell lung cancers.[19,20]

Because of the many steps involved in the PI3K-Akt pathway, there are many approaches for the treatment of neuroendocrine malignancies. Two PI3K inhibitors, LY294002 and wortmannin, have been studied in human cancer cells, but LY294002 has been examined in detail as a potential therapy for gastrointestinal and pulmonary carcinoids as well as small cell lung cancers. These inhibitors specifically target the p110 subunit. Krystal and colleagues[4] found that treatment with a PI3K inhibitor led to decreased growth and apoptosis of small cell lung cancer cells, but more importantly, it increased the sensitivity of the cells to etoposide chemotherapy. In a pulmonary carcinoid cell line, treatment with LY294002 led to decreased growth of cancer cells as well as decreased expression of the NET markers, achaete-scute complex-like (ASCL) 1 and CgA.[16] Similar findings have been discovered in gastrointestinal carcinoid cells.[5]

One of the downstream targets of both the PI3K-Akt and Ras/Raf/MEK/ERK pathways, mTOR has been a focus in the treatment of NETs. mTOR is a serine/threonine kinase that regulates cell proliferation and apoptosis, and treatment of carcinoid cells with the mTOR inhibitor, rapamycin, has been shown to decrease tumor growth both in vitro and in vivo.[21] Two rapamycin derivatives, temsirolimus and everolimus, have been tested in multicenter phase 2 clinical trials on patients with NETs with some promising results. In the initial studies published on temsirolimus, 63.9% of patients had either a partial response to treatment or stable disease for at least 2 months.[22] The everolimus study had similar initial results, with 92% of patients having stable disease or a partial response to treatment.[23] Based on these findings, further clinical trials of these compounds are ongoing.

Another important downstream target of the PI3K-Akt and Ras/Raf/MEK/ERK pathways is GSK-3β, a serine/threonine protein kinase, also found to regulate multiple cellular processes such as metabolism, proliferation, and survival.[24] Studies have demonstrated that unlike most kinases, GSK-3β is active in the non-phosphorylated state and becomes inhibited when phosphorylated.[25] Inhibition of GSK-3β has been shown to decrease tumor growth in several cancers, including pancreas, colon, and prostate cancers. Kunnimalaiyaan and colleagues[26] first demonstrated that treatment with a GSK-3β inhibitor, such as lithium chloride, a Food and Drug Administration (FDA)-approved medication in the treatment of bipolar disorder, reduced the expression of ASCL1 and CgA in medullary thyroid cancer cells. This study also suggested that lithium chloride induces cell growth inhibition in vitro and in vivo via cell cycle arrest. This finding led to a phase 2 trial of lithium chloride for the treatment of medullary thyroid cancer, which is currently underway.

THE NOTCH1 SIGNALING PATHWAY

The Notch1 signaling pathway regulates cellular differentiation, proliferation, and cell survival. Notch1 has 5 ligands, referred to as deltalike ligands (DLL-1, DLL-3, DLL-4, JAG-1, and JAG-2).[27] Notch1 is a transmembrane receptor having an N-terminal extracellular domain with epidermal growth factor–like repeats that mediate ligand binding (**Fig. 2**).[28] In the absence of ligand binding, an area of 3 cysteine-rich Notch/Lin-12 repeats on the extracellular domain interacts to prevent signaling.[28] Once a ligand binds to the Notch1 receptor, 2 proteolytic cleavages occur, releasing the Notch1 intracellular domain (NICD).[29] The NICD translocates to the nucleus and binds to a transactivation complex known as DNA-binding protein complex CSL (C promoter–binding factor 1 [CBF-1], suppressor of hairless, and Lag-1). This binding results in the activation of multiple target genes such as hairy enhancer of split 1 (HES-1), which in turn controls the expression of ASCL1.[27] ASCL1 has been shown to play a role in the development of pulmonary neuroendocrine cells, thyroid C cells, and adrenal chromaffin cells, and its levels are decreased when Notch signaling is active.[30,31]

The Notch1 signaling pathway was initially identified as being oncogenic in human T-cell malignancies.[32] This pathway was then found to be upregulated in many different cancers, including pancreatic cancer, colon cancer, cervical cancer, ovarian cancer, and renal cell carcinoma.[7,8] In contrast, researchers have demonstrated minimal or absent Notch1 signaling in prostate cancer and in NETs such as carcinoid, small cell lung, and medullary thyroid cancers, suggesting its role as a tumor suppressor.[9–11] As expected, with minimal Notch1 signaling present, these cancer

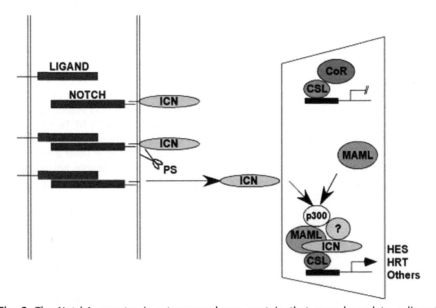

Fig. 2. The Notch1 receptor is a transmembrane protein that once bound to a ligand undergoes cleavage releasing the Notch intracellular domain (ICN). ICN migrates to the nucleus and forms a DNA-binding protein complex CSL (C promoter–binding factor 1 [CBF-1], suppressor of hairless, and Lag-1), resulting in the activation of multiple target genes including hairy enhancer of split (HES). CoR, nuclear receptor corepressor; HRT, hairy-related transcription factors; MAML, mastermind-like proteins. (*From* Maillard I, Pear W. Notch and cancer: best to avoid the ups and downs. Cancer Cell 2003;3(3):204; with permission.)

cells express high levels of ASCL1, which make it useful as a NET marker. Nakakura and colleagues[10] treated pancreatic carcinoid cells with a Notch1 viral vector. After treatment, cellular growth was suppressed and there was increased expression of HES-1 and decreased expressions of ASCL1, CgA, NSE, and synaptophysin. Similarly, treatment of a small cell lung cancer cell line with a Notch1 viral vector led to a reduction in the levels of NET markers as well as growth suppression of these cells.[33] In another study of medullary thyroid cancer by Kunnimalaiyaan and colleagues,[34] a medullary thyroid cancer cell line was treated with a doxycycline-inducible Notch1 plasmid. HES-1 proteins levels were increased, while levels of ASCL1 and calcitonin were decreased, correlating with the amount of Notch1 present in these cells.

Although demonstrating Notch1 as a tumor suppressor in NETs has been successful, the discovery of Notch1 activating agents has been more difficult. In 2005, Stockhausen and colleagues[35] demonstrated that valproic acid (VPA), a histone deacetylase (HDAC) inhibitor, increased Notch1 protein levels in neuroblastoma cells. Based on this work, studies were undertaken into the role that VPA could play in both pulmonary and gastrointestinal carcinoid cells. VPA was successful in inhibiting NET cell growth via G1 phase cell cycle arrest and suppressing expression of tumor markers both in vitro and in vivo.[36] Other HDAC inhibitors such as suberoyl bishydroxamic acid have also demonstrated Notch1 activation and NET suppression.[37] Given these promising results, phase 2 trials testing HDAC inhibitors as Notch1–activating compounds are currently underway.

RAS/RAF/MEK/ERK PATHWAY

The Ras/Raf/MEK/ERK pathway begins with Ras, a G protein. Ras is activated on phosphorylation of a GDP, which then activates Raf, a family of 3 cytosolic kinases, of which Raf-1 is the most important in cell differentiation (**Fig. 3**).[12] Once Raf is activated, it causes further downstream activation of MEK and ERK. This pathway plays an integral role in cell differentiation, growth, and survival.[38,39]

Mutations in Ras and Raf lead to overexpression of this pathway and tumorigenesis in colon, lung, and many pancreatic cancers.[40] Conversely, the Ras/Raf/MEK/ERK pathway has been shown to be minimally active or absent in NETs such as small cell lung cancers, carcinoids, and medullary thyroid cancer.[41–43] Small cell lung cancer cells transfected with a Raf-1 construct demonstrated increased Raf-1 activity and decreased cellular growth, suggesting that the Ras/Raf pathway could function as a tumor suppressor.[41,42] In similar experiments on pancreatic carcinoid cells, researchers were able to demonstrate a reduction in levels of 5-HT and CgA with the activation of Raf-1.[43,44] In medullary thyroid cancer, activation of Raf-1 has led not only to growth suppression and a reduction in the neuroendocrine hormones, 5-HT and calcitonin, but also to reduced levels of the RET proto-oncogene.[11,45] This effect of activation of Raf-1 is evidence that the Ras/Raf/MEK/ERK pathway may play a role in NET suppression not only via auto activation but also by interactions with other signaling pathways.

Given the decreased expression of the Ras/Raf/MEK/ERK pathway in NETs and decrease in cell growth and hormone secretion with Raf-1 activation, targeting this pathway may serve as a potential therapeutic option. One compound ZM336372 was initially found to cause Raf-1 inhibition but demonstrated a significant increase in Raf-1 activation in vitro.[46] When pancreatic and pulmonary carcinoid cells were treated with the agent, there was an increase in Raf-1 and ERK phosphorylation and a reduction in cell growth and hormone production.[47] In vivo studies of ZM336372 have not yet been undertaken because of its insolubility at high doses. Therefore, other Raf-1 activators

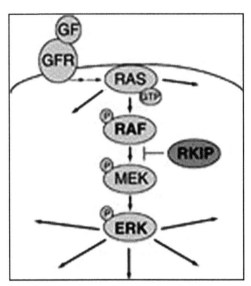

Fig. 3. RAS, an intracellular G protein, is phosphorylated, leading to the activation of RAF. Once RAF is activated, it in turn phosphorylates MEK, which in turn phosphorylates and activates the ERK. Once activated, ERK phosphorylates cytoplasmic proteins and translocates into the nucleus, where it regulates transcription of genes involved in cell differentiation, proliferation, and survival. GF, growth factor, GFR, growth factor receptor; P, phosphate; RKIP, Raf kinase inhibitor protein. (*From* Houben R, Michel B, Vetter-Kauczok C, et al. Absence of classical MAP kinase pathway signalling in Merkel cell carcinoma. J Invest Dermatol 2006;126(5):1136; with permission.)

such as tautomycin, a potent and specific protein phosphatase inhibitor isolated from *Streptomyces spiroverticillatus*, have been studied. In 2008, Pinchot and colleagues[48] reported that low doses of tautomycin inhibited proliferation of carcinoid cells and suppressed CgA and ASCL1 via cell cycle arrest. Further testing of tautomycin in vivo is needed, but clinical trials of streptozocin, a related compound, used to treat pancreatic islet cell tumors is underway in carcinoids.[49] Leflunomide, an FDA-approved rheumatoid arthritis medication, has also shown promise as a treatment of NETs via Raf-1 activation. In a study by Cook and colleagues,[50] leflunomide and its active metabolite, teriflunomide, were shown to decrease the expression of NET markers and to inhibit in vitro and in vivo carcinoid cell proliferation. These studies demonstrate the potential of future treatments of NETs via targeting of the Ras/Raf/MEK/ERK pathway.

THE RET PATHWAY

The RET gene encodes a tyrosine kinase receptor, which is a single transmembrane receptor with a cysteine-rich extracellular domain and 2 intracellular tyrosine kinase subdomains.[51] Several previously discussed pathways such as PI3K-Akt and Ras/Raf/ERK/MEK have been known to interact with the RET pathway.[52] Other downstream targets linked to the RET tyrosine kinase receptor include mitogen-activated protein kinase (MAPK), fibroblast growth factor receptor substrate 2, and phosphoinositide-dependent kinase 5.[53] Through all of these various targets, RET plays important roles in cell differentiation, growth, and survival.

Multiple mutations in the RET receptor are responsible for the development of medullary thyroid cancer. In familial medullary thyroid cancers associated with

MEN2A, mutations causing the unpairing of cysteine residues in the extracellular domain are responsible for the activation of RET kinase.[54] Conversely, a mutation of the intracellular domain is responsible for the development of familial medullary thyroid cancers associated with MEN2B.[54] Somatic mutations of RET have also been discovered in sporadic medullary thyroid cancers.

Several tyrosine kinase inhibitors directed at RET kinase have been tested to treat medullary thyroid cancer. Vandetanib is a tyrosine kinase inhibitor that also inhibits vascular endothelial growth factor receptor 2.[55] Vandetanib has been shown to block phosphorylation in the most common MEN2A and MEN2B mutations.[56] A phase 2 clinical trial of vandetanib in patients with metastatic familial medullary thyroid carcinoma demonstrated partial response or stable disease in 40% of patients at 24 weeks.[57] Sunitinib is another promising tyrosine kinase inhibitor that affects angiogenesis as well as directly inhibits cellular proliferation via both the vascular endothelial growth factor and the RET pathways.[22,58] Patients with advanced pancreatic NETs treated with sunitinib demonstrated increased median progression-free survival as well as an overall response rate of 9.3%, with stable disease reported in 34.9% of patients.[59] Further clinical trials of these and other RET tyrosine kinase receptors are ongoing.

SUMMARY

The development, growth, and survival of NETs depend on a variety of complex signaling mechanisms. Extensive research has begun to elucidate the details of the multiple pathways that play fundamental roles in carcinoids, small cell lung cancers, and medullary thyroid cancer, and continued efforts into understanding the interactions of these pathways are imperative. Many therapeutic compounds have now shown promise in the treatment and palliation of NETs, but further research into definitive medical therapies is needed.

REFERENCES

1. Kim T, Grobmyer S, Liu C, et al. Primary presacral neuroendocrine tumor associated with imperforate anus. World J Surg Oncol 2007;5:115.
2. Luo J, Manning B, Cantley L. Targeting the PI3K-Akt pathway in human cancer: rationale and promise. Cancer Cell 2003;4(4):257–62.
3. Vivanco I, Sawyers C. The phosphatidylinositol 3-kinase AKT pathway in human cancer. Nat Rev Cancer 2002;2(7):489–501.
4. Krystal G, Sulanke G, Litz J. Inhibition of phosphatidylinositol 3-kinase-Akt signaling blocks growth, promotes apoptosis, and enhances sensitivity of small cell lung cancer cells to chemotherapy. Mol Cancer Ther 2002;1(11):913–22.
5. Pitt S, Chen H, Kunnimalaiyaan M. Inhibition of phosphatidylinositol 3-kinase/Akt signaling suppresses tumor cell proliferation and neuroendocrine marker expression in GI carcinoid tumors. Ann Surg Oncol 2009;16(10):2936–42.
6. Murtaugh L, Stanger B, Kwan K, et al. Notch signaling controls multiple steps of pancreatic differentiation. Proc Natl Acad Sci U S A 2003;100(25):14920–5.
7. Kadesch T. Notch signaling: the demise of elegant simplicity. Curr Opin Genet Dev 2004;14(5):506–12.
8. Radtke F, Raj K. The role of Notch in tumorigenesis: oncogene or tumour suppressor? Nat Rev Cancer 2003;3(10):756–67.
9. Kunnimalaiyaan M, Traeger K, Chen H. Conservation of the Notch1 signaling pathway in gastrointestinal carcinoid cells. Am J Physiol Gastrointest Liver Physiol 2005;289(4):G636–42.

10. Nakakura E, Sriuranpong V, Kunnimalaiyaan M, et al. Regulation of neuroendocrine differentiation in gastrointestinal carcinoid tumor cells by Notch signaling. J Clin Endocrinol Metab 2005;90(7):4350–6.

11. Sippel R, Carpenter J, Kunnimalaiyaan M, et al. The role of human achaete-scute homolog-1 in medullary thyroid cancer cells. Surgery 2003;134(6):866–71 [discussion: 871–3].

12. Kunnimalaiyaan M, Chen H. The Raf-1 pathway: a molecular target for treatment of select neuroendocrine tumors? Anticancer Drugs 2006;17(2):139–42.

13. Greco A, Borrello M, Miranda C, et al. Molecular pathology of differentiated thyroid cancer. Q J Nucl Med Mol Imaging 2009;53(5):440–53.

14. Walker G, Hayward N. Pathways to melanoma development: lessons from the mouse. J Invest Dermatol 2002;119(4):783–92.

15. Zarebczan B, Chen H. Multi-targeted approach in the treatment of thyroid cancer. Minerva Chir 2010;65(1):59–69.

16. Pitt S, Chen H, Kunnimalaiyaan M. Phosphatidylinositol 3-kinase-Akt signaling in pulmonary carcinoid cells. J Am Coll Surg 2009;209(1):82–8.

17. Wang L, Ignat A, Axiotis C. Differential expression of the PTEN tumor suppressor protein in fetal and adult neuroendocrine tissues and tumors: progressive loss of PTEN expression in poorly differentiated neuroendocrine neoplasms. Appl Immunohistochem Mol Morphol 2002;10(2):139–46.

18. Shah T, Hochhauser D, Frow R, et al. Epidermal growth factor receptor expression and activation in neuroendocrine tumours. J Neuroendocrinol 2006;18(5):355–60.

19. Forgacs E, Biesterveld E, Sekido Y, et al. Mutation analysis of the PTEN/MMAC1 gene in lung cancer. Oncogene 1998;17(12):1557–65.

20. Yokomizo A, Tindall D, Drabkin H, et al. PTEN/MMAC1 mutations identified in small cell, but not in non-small cell lung cancers. Oncogene 1998;17(4):475–9.

21. Moreno A, Akcakanat A, Munsell M, et al. Antitumor activity of rapamycin and octreotide as single agents or in combination in neuroendocrine tumors. Endocr Relat Cancer 2008;15(1):257–66.

22. Duran I, Kortmansky J, Singh D, et al. A phase II clinical and pharmacodynamic study of temsirolimus in advanced neuroendocrine carcinomas. Br J Cancer 2006;95(9):1148–54.

23. Yao J, Phan A, Chang D, et al. Efficacy of RAD001 (everolimus) and octreotide LAR in advanced low- to intermediate-grade neuroendocrine tumors: results of a phase II study. J Clin Oncol 2008;26(26):4311–8.

24. Hardt S, Sadoshima J. Glycogen synthase kinase-3beta: a novel regulator of cardiac hypertrophy and development. Circ Res 2002;90(10):1055–63.

25. Cohen P, Frame S. The renaissance of GSK3. Nat Rev Mol Cell Biol 2001;2(10):769–76.

26. Kunnimalaiyaan M, Vaccaro A, Ndiaye M, et al. Inactivation of glycogen synthase kinase-3beta, a downstream target of the raf-1 pathway, is associated with growth suppression in medullary thyroid cancer cells. Mol Cancer Ther 2007;6(3):1151–8.

27. Cook M, Yu X, Chen H. Notch in the development of thyroid C-cells and the treatment of medullary thyroid cancer. Am J Transl Res 2010;2(1):119–25.

28. Kunnimalaiyaan M, Chen H. Tumor suppressor role of Notch-1 signaling in neuroendocrine tumors. Oncologist 2007;12(5):535–42.

29. Allenspach E, Maillard I, Aster J, et al. Notch signaling in cancer. Cancer Biol Ther 2002;1(5):466–76.

30. Ito T, Udaka N, Yazawa T, et al. Basic helix-loop-helix transcription factors regulate the neuroendocrine differentiation of fetal mouse pulmonary epithelium. Development 2000;127(18):3913–21.
31. Lanigan T, DeRaad S, Russo A. Requirement of the MASH-1 transcription factor for neuroendocrine differentiation of thyroid C cells. J Neurobiol 1998;34(2): 126–34.
32. Ellisen L, Bird J, West D, et al. TAN-1, the human homolog of the Drosophila Notch gene, is broken by chromosomal translocations in T lymphoblastic neoplasms. Cell 1991;66(4):649–61.
33. Sriuranpong V, Borges M, Ravi R, et al. Notch signaling induces cell cycle arrest in small cell lung cancer cells. Cancer Res 2001;61(7):3200–5.
34. Kunnimalaiyaan M, Vaccaro A, Ndiaye M, et al. Overexpression of the NOTCH1 intracellular domain inhibits cell proliferation and alters the neuroendocrine phenotype of medullary thyroid cancer cells. J Biol Chem 2006;281(52): 39819–30.
35. Stockhausen M, Sjölund J, Manetopoulos C, et al. Effects of the histone deacetylase inhibitor valproic acid on notch signalling in human neuroblastoma cells. Br J Cancer 2005;92(4):751–9.
36. Greenblatt D, Vaccaro A, Jaskula-Sztul R, et al. Valproic acid activates Notch-1 signaling and regulates the neuroendocrine phenotype in carcinoid cancer cells. Oncologist 2007;12(8):942–51.
37. Ning L, Greenblatt D, Kunnimalaiyaan M, et al. Suberoyl bis-hydroxamic acid activates Notch-1 signaling and induces apoptosis in medullary thyroid carcinoma cells. Oncologist 2008;13(2):98–104.
38. Chen H, Kunnimalaiyaan M, Van Gompel J. Medullary thyroid cancer: the functions of raf-1 and human achaete-scute homologue-1. Thyroid 2005;15(6): 511–21.
39. Dhillon A, Kolch W. Oncogenic B-Raf mutations: crystal clear at last. Cancer Cell 2004;5(4):303–4.
40. Younes N, Fulton N, Tanaka R, et al. The presence of K-12 ras mutations in duodenal adenocarcinomas and the absence of ras mutations in other small bowel adenocarcinomas and carcinoid tumors. Cancer 1997;79(9):1804–8.
41. Ravi R, Thiagalingam A, Weber E, et al. Raf-1 causes growth suppression and alteration of neuroendocrine markers in DMS53 human small-cell lung cancer cells. Am J Respir Cell Mol Biol 1999;20(4):543–9.
42. Ravi R, Weber E, McMahon M, et al. Activated Raf-1 causes growth arrest in human small cell lung cancer cells. J Clin Invest 1998;101(1):153–9.
43. Sippel R, Carpenter J, Kunnimalaiyaan M, et al. Raf-1 activation suppresses neuroendocrine marker and hormone levels in human gastrointestinal carcinoid cells. Am J Physiol Gastrointest Liver Physiol 2003;285(2):G245–54.
44. Sippel R, Chen H. Activation of the ras/raf-1 signal transduction pathway in carcinoid tumor cells results in morphologic transdifferentiation. Surgery 2002;132(6): 1035–9 [discussion: 1039].
45. Park J, Strock C, Ball D, et al. The Ras/Raf/MEK/extracellular signal-regulated kinase pathway induces autocrine-paracrine growth inhibition via the leukemia inhibitory factor/JAK/STAT pathway. Mol Cell Biol 2003;23(2):543–54.
46. Hall-Jackson C, Eyers P, Cohen P, et al. Paradoxical activation of Raf by a novel Raf inhibitor. Chem Biol 1999;6(8):559–68.
47. Van Gompel J, Kunnimalaiyaan M, Holen K, et al. ZM336372, a Raf-1 activator, suppresses growth and neuroendocrine hormone levels in carcinoid tumor cells. Mol Cancer Ther 2005;4(6):910–7.

48. Pinchot S, Adler J, Luo Y, et al. Tautomycin suppresses growth and neuroendocrine hormone markers in carcinoid cells through activation of the Raf-1 pathway. Am J Surg 2009;197(3):313–9.

49. ClinicalTrials.gov. Available at: http://clinicaltrials.gov/ct2/show/NCT00602082?term=streptozocin&rank=2. Accessed April 20, 2010.

50. Cook M, Pinchot S, Jaskula-Sztul R, et al. Identification of a novel Raf-1 pathway activator that inhibits gastrointestinal carcinoid cell growth. Mol Cancer Ther 2010;9(2):429–37.

51. Cakir M, Grossman A. Medullary thyroid cancer: molecular biology and novel molecular therapies. Neuroendocrinology 2009;90(4):323–48.

52. de Groot J, Links T, Plukker J, et al. RET as a diagnostic and therapeutic target in sporadic and hereditary endocrine tumors. Endocr Rev 2006;27(5):535–60.

53. Segouffin-Cariou C, Billaud M. Transforming ability of MEN2A-RET requires activation of the phosphatidylinositol 3-kinase/AKT signaling pathway. J Biol Chem 2000;275(5):3568–76.

54. Santoro M, Melillo R, Carlomagno F, et al. Molecular biology of the MEN2 gene. J Intern Med 1998;243(6):505–8.

55. Herbst R, Heymach J, O'Reilly M, et al. Vandetanib (ZD6474): an orally available receptor tyrosine kinase inhibitor that selectively targets pathways critical for tumor growth and angiogenesis. Expert Opin Investig Drugs 2007;16(2):239–49.

56. Carlomagno F, Vitagliano D, Guida T, et al. ZD6474, an orally available inhibitor of KDR tyrosine kinase activity, efficiently blocks oncogenic RET kinases. Cancer Res 2002;62(24):7284–90.

57. Sherman S. Early clinical studies of novel therapies for thyroid cancers. Endocrinol Metab Clin North Am 2008;37(2):511–24.

58. Kulke M, Scherübl H. Accomplishments in 2008 in the management of gastrointestinal neuroendocrine tumors. Gastrointest Cancer Res 2009;3(5 Suppl 2): S62–6.

59. Dimou A, Syrigos K, Saif M. Neuroendocrine tumors of the pancreas: what's new. Highlights from the "2010 ASCO Gastrointestinal Cancers Symposium". Orlando, FL, USA. January 22–24, 2010. JOP 2010;11(2):135–8.

Novel Anticancer Agents in Clinical Trials for Well-Differentiated Neuroendocrine Tumors

Sandrine Faivre, MD, PhD, Marie-Paule Sablin, MD,
Chantal Dreyer, MD, Eric Raymond, MD, PhD*

KEYWORDS

- Sunitinib • Everolimus • Bevacizumab • Carcinoid
- Angiogenesis • mTOR inhibitors

Neuroendocrine tumors (NETs) are rare malignancies that arise from endocrine cells located in various anatomic locations. Incidence of these tumors has dramatically increased during the last 30 years, currently ranking 2.5 to 5 per 100,000 inhabitants in the United States.[1,2] NETs developing from the aerodigestive tract are also named carcinoid tumors, whereas tumors of the endocrine tissues of the pancreas are known as pancreatic NETs (PNETs) or islet cell carcinomas. The degree of differentiation plays an important role in the therapeutic approaches of NETs.[3,4] Although sometimes heterogeneous, well-differentiated and poorly differentiated/high-grade NETs are grouped based on the expression of synaptophysin and chromogranin that are detected by immunohistochemistry; they display different biologic and clinical behaviors and strikingly different sensitivity to systemic therapies.[5–8] High-grade

Information for this review was compiled by searching PubMed and MEDLINE databases for articles published until January 2010. Only articles published in English were considered. The search terms used included neuroendocrine tumor in association with the search terms angiogenesis, VEGFR, PDGFR, sunitinib, sorafenib, bevacizumab, thalidomide, mTOR inhibintors, rapamycin, rapalogues, temozolomide, streptozotocin, somatostatin analogs, IGF1-R inhibitor, natural product, metastatic, clinical trial, islet cell carcinomas, carcinoid tumors, targeted therapy, cytotoxic therapy, and prognosis. Full articles were obtained, and references were checked for additional material when appropriate.

This work was supported in part by the Association d'Aide à la Recherche et à l'Enseignement en Cancérologie (AAREC), Clichy, France.

Department of Medical Oncology, Beaujon University Hospital (AP-HP, Paris 7 Diderot), Clichy, France

* Corresponding author. Department of Medical Oncology (INSERM U728, Paris 7), Beaujon University Hospital, Assistance Publique, Hôpitaux de Paris, 100 Boulevard du Général Leclerc, 92110 Clichy, France.

E-mail address: eric.raymond@bjn.aphp.fr

Endocrinol Metab Clin N Am 39 (2010) 811–826
doi:10.1016/j.ecl.2010.09.006
0889-8529/10/$ – see front matter © 2010 Elsevier Inc. All rights reserved.

endo.theclinics.com

NETs seem to be driven by a high proliferation rate as reflected by the high expression of Ki67 (MIB) and are thus closely related to aggressive pulmonary small cell carcinomas, whereas well-differentiated NETs seem to primarily depend on tumor angiogenesis, as demonstrated by a high level of microvessel density with a more indolent clinical behavior.[9,10] Thereby, sensitivity of well-differentiated NETs to cytotoxic chemotherapy seems to be erratic, whereas treatment of advanced poorly differentiated NETs relies on antiproliferative drugs and currently derives from small cell lung carcinomas and consists of cisplatin-etoposide (VePeside) combination chemotherapy.[11]

Surgery remains the mainstay of curative treatment of patients with resectable well-differentiated NETs.[12] However, most patients with NETs are not amenable to curative resection because of multiple hepatic, lung, or bone metastasis at the time of primary diagnosis or recurrence. Chemoembolization, radiofrequency ablation, or percutaneous ethanol injection are locoregional treatments that may offer palliative benefits for those with metastasis primarily located in the liver.[13,14] For patients with bulky liver involvement, rapid tumor progression, or extrahepatic spread, chemotherapy has been offered as a palliative approach, aiming at delaying tumor-related symptoms and tumor progression and improving overall survival.[15] Cancer cell proliferation is highly variable in well-differentiated NETs as reflected by variable mitotic indexes and various levels of Ki67 expression. Variability in cancer cell proliferation may have accounted for the inconsistent results using chemotherapy in well-differentiated NETs; a trend toward a better benefit using chemotherapy was observed in patients with tumors with high mitotic index and Ki67 levels higher than 2%. So far, the only chemotherapy licensed for use in PNETs is streptozotocin, a DNA alkylating agent that displays high toxicity for islet cells and depends on several DNA repair mechanisms for cytotoxicity. Other drugs are doxorubicin and 5-fluorouracil, which, when combined with streptozotocin, demonstrated encouraging results in clinical trials reported by Moertel and colleagues[16,17] and Kouvaraki and colleagues[18] in the late 1980s. However, the initially reported response rates of up to 69% with doxorubicin-streptozotocin combinations have recently been challenged in clinical trials using modern imaging techniques and efficacy criteria, suggesting that the magnitude of clinical benefit using streptozotocin-based chemotherapy may have been previously overestimated.[19,20]

Thus, new treatment options are required for subjects with unresectable PNETs. Novel targeted therapies have yielded significant clinical improvements in the treatment of various malignancies. Consistent preclinical data on cell signaling pathways involved in endocrine tumors have led to the identification of several drug targets, providing a rationale for clinical investigations of targeted therapies in well-differentiated NETs. Until recently, clinical experiences with novel anticancer agents in NETs derived primarily from uncontrolled phase 2 studies with limited number of patients. The lack of a control group and selection bias that are frequently associated with small phase 2 trials often led to inconsistent results and have made difficult assessing the benefit derived from novel therapies in patients with NETs. Efforts were newly made by cooperative groups and industrial sponsors to design cooperative trials, allowing performing large randomized trials in these rare tumors. This approach generated more robust data and steady progresses.

This review primarily focuses on recent advances in well-differentiated NETs and breakthroughs that have been made in clinical trials. Ongoing clinical trials are displayed in **Table 1** (http://www.clinicaltrial.gov).

Table 1
Clinical trials using anticancer agents in patients with gastrointestinal neuroendocrine tumors

Type of Drugs	Clinical Stage	Indications
Somatostatin-derived Compounds		
Pentetreotide In 111	Phase 2	Neuroendocrine
Lanreotide autogel	Phase 3	Enteropancreatic endocrine tumors
Pasireotide long-acting release vs octreotide long-acting release	Phase 3	Metastatic carcinoid tumors
Lanreotide injection	Phase 3	Carcinoid syndrome
Depot ocreotide with either interferon-α2b or bevacizumab	Phase 3	Carcinoid tumors
LX1606	Phase 2	Carcinoid syndrome
Yittrium Y 90-DOTA-tyr3-ocreotide	Phase I	Pediatric patients aged 2–25 years with somatostatin receptor positive tumors
IGF1-R Inhibitors		
IMC-A12 combination with octreotide depot	Phase 2	Carcinoids and PNETs
AMG479	Phase 2	Carcinoid and PNETs
Antiangiogenic Agents		
Bevacizumab with chemotherapy	Phase 1/2	NETs
PTK787/ZK222584	Phase 2	NETs
EGFR inhibitors		
Erlotinib and pertuzumab	Phase 2	NETs
mTOR Inhibitors		
Everolimus with erlotinib	Phase 2	NETs
Everolimus and pasireotide	Phase 1	NETs
Everolimus and sorafenib	Phase 1	NETS
Everolimus and temozolomide	Phase 1/2	Carcinoids and PNETs
Temsirolimus and bevacizumab	Phase 2	Carcinoids and PNETs
Chemotherapy		
Capecitabine and temozolomide	Phase 2	NETs
PVA microporous hydrosphere of doxorubicin	Phase 1	NETs
Miscellaneous		
Lithium	Phase 2	Low-grade NETs
BB-10901 (CD56 inhibitor)	Phase 1	Carcinoid tumors
Yttrium 90 glass microsphere	Phase 1/2	Various, including endocrine tumors

Data from www.cancer.gov (Accessed date May 1, 2010).

SOMATOSTATIN ANALOGUES AND RADIOLABELED NUCLEOTIDES

Somatostatin is a 14-amino-acid-long peptide that regulates the secretion of the growth hormone, insulin, glucagon, and gastrin.[21] About 80% of carcinoid tumors express somatostatin receptors. Somatostatin and somatostatin receptors have been the only relevant targets for a long period before the identification of novel molecular drug targets, such as vascular endothelial growth factor (VEGF) receptor (VEGFR), *platelet-derived growth factor (PDGF) receptor* (PDGFR), and mammalian target of rapamycin (mTOR), which are described later in the article.[22,23]

Octreotide is a synthetic 8-amino-acid-long analogue of somatostatin designed to bind with high-affinity somatostatin receptors.[24] Depot, long-acting release somatostatin analogues have recently been developed, allowing once-monthly intramuscular injections. Somatostatin analogues were initially used to inhibit clinical symptoms associated with the endocrine secretion of hormones in carcinoid tumors (carcinoid syndrome) and secreting PNETs. Laboratory data also suggested that some well-differentiated NETs may express somatostatin receptors and may depend on autocrine somatostatin activation for tumor growth. Consistently, demonstration of disease stabilization has been reported in some patients with progressive disease when treated with octreotide and lanreotide. Thus, somatostatin analogues have been proposed to control the growth of tumors in patients with NETs. Until recently, the lack of large phase 2 trials or randomized studies has made difficult the appraisal of the real therapeutic benefit for those therapeutic approaches. The first placebo-controlled, double-blind, phase 3 study on the effect of long-acting release octreotide in the control of tumor growth in patients with well-differentiated metastatic midgut NETs has been reported recently.[25] The median time to tumor progression in the octreotide and placebo groups was 14.3 and 6 months (hazard ratio [HR], 0.34; P = .000072), respectively. However, the benefit of somatostatin analogues in this trial seems to be limited to patients with less than 10% tumor liver involvement and in patients with surgically removed primary tumors. The efficacy of octreotide in patients with large tumor burden and nonresectable primary tumors remains uncertain. Furthermore, data provided in this trial did not report information on tumor progression at study entry, making difficult to identify the subset of patients who may benefit the most from this therapy. A similar multicenter, placebo-controlled European phase 3 study is underway to assess whether lanreotide autogel prolongs time to disease progression in patients with nonfunctioning PNETs (www.clinicaltrials.gov). Taken together, these recent data suggest that patients with symptoms resulting from hypersecretion of peptides and hormones may achieve improved symptom control and delayed progression from somatostatin analogues in 35% to 70% of cases,[22,24] although objective radiologic responses are usually less than 5%.[23,25] Subgroups of patients who may benefit from cytostatic effects of somatostatin analogues remain to be identified but are likely to be limited to a subset of patients with low tumor burden, resected primary tumor, and slowly progressive disease, which unfortunately are infrequent criteria for advanced NETs. Antitumor activity has been reported with investigational somatostatin analogues, and combination with interferon (IFN)-α seemed to offer limited additional benefit.[26]

Several radioisotope-linked somatostatin analogues have been investigated during the past 10 years, including Indium 111, Yttrium 90, and Lutetium 177.[27,28] The basic principle of this approach lies in using high-energy beta-particle emitters to generate radiation-induced DNA damages in somatostatin-targeted carcinoma cells. Most reported clinical data are derived from small phase 2 trials, making it difficult to address the overall clinical advantage of these approaches over other medical treatments. Studies of the Yttrium 90–labeled somatostatin analogue reported response rates of up to 27%.[29,30] The European Multicenter Analysis of a Universal Receptor Imaging and Treatment Initiative used lanreotide Y 90 to evaluate 39 patients with NETs.[31] Minor tumor regressions were seen in 20% of patients, and 44% of patients achieved stable disease. Adverse effects associated with octreotide Y 90 include renal and hematologic toxicities. A more extensive somewhat retrospective cohort analysis of 504 patients with metastatic NETs who received octreotate Lu 177 was reported in 2008.[32] There was complete response in 2% of the patients, partial response in 28%, and minor response in 16%. The median time to progression was approximately 40 months, but only 43% of patients had documented disease progression before study entry. Serious adverse events consisted of myelodysplastic syndrome and liver toxicity. Theoretically, cancer cells that are likely to be affected by this approach should express somatostatin receptors and lack DNA repair mechanisms involved in radiation resistance. From a biologic standpoint, it would be more interesting to investigate the expression in NET of main DNA repair mechanisms classically involved in beta-emitter radiation-induced DNA damages to identify patients with tumor types that are more likely to respond to this approach. In addition, randomized controlled trials with well-defined inclusion criteria are urgently needed to define the real benefit and safety of this approach in NETs. Until then, the use of radiolabeled somatostatin analogues cannot be considered as a standard treatment of NETs and shall remain an investigational approach within the frames of clinical studies or companionate administrations for patients who failed prior registered treatments.

NOVEL TARGETS IN ANGIOGENESIS AND CELL SIGNALING

As alluded earlier, somatostatin and somatostatin receptors that belong to the G-protein–coupled receptor family and tyrosine kinase receptors, such as insulin-like growth factor (IGF) 1 receptor (IGF1-R), have been shown to be capable of controlling cell proliferation in NETs. In addition, other cells such as endothelial cells and pericytes were shown to play an important role in the development and the maintenance of blood supply for proliferating cancer cells through the development of tumor angiogenesis (**Fig. 1**). As such, VEGF and VEGFR have been shown as major players involved in the endothelial cell survival, whereas PDGF and PDGFR have been considered as important stimulating factors for pericytes functions.[33–36] Downstream cell signaling may vary from one model to another, but 4 major cell signaling pathways have been shown to stimulate cellular proliferation and survival for cancer cell proliferation and angiogenesis. The phosphoinositide 3-kinase (PI3k)/AKT/mTOR and the phospholipaseC/protein kinase C pathways seemed crucial for downstream VEGFR and PDGFR signaling. The PI3k/AKT/mTOR as well as the RAS/RAF/MAPK pathways are important in signal transduction of IGF1-R. Finally, the PI3k/AKT/mTOR and the JAK/STAT pathways were shown to control signal transduction induced by somatostatin receptors. At the molecular level, some degree of redundancy may exist between these cell-signaling pathways and may account for the lack of activity of inhibitors inhibiting one of those targets with a high level of specificity. As shown in **Fig. 2**, hypoxia occurring in tumors that reach a certain volume seems to be the main driving force for hypoxia-inducible factor (HIF)-1 and HIF-2 expression, leading to VEGF and PDGF secretion by cancer cells.[9] Whereas VEGF directly attracts and stimulates the proliferation of endothelial cells, PDGF stimulates the proliferation of pericytes, leading to the development of tumor angiogenesis. Novel anticancer agents such as sunitinib eventually block the activation of VEGFR and PDGFR, inducing apoptosis in endothelial cells and pericytes and thereby inhibiting angiogenesis (**Fig. 3**). mTOR inhibitors currently

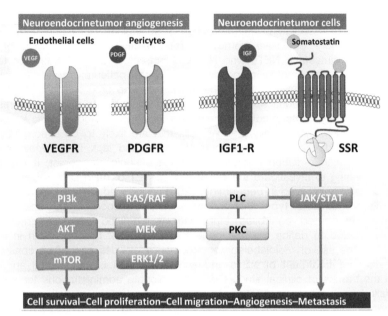

Fig. 1. Main receptors and transduction pathways involved in signaling of cancer cells and angiogenesis in neuroendocrine tumors. mTOR, mammalian target of rapamycin; PDGF, platelet derived growth factors; PDGFR, platelet derived growth receptors; PKC, protein kinase C; PLC, phospholipase C; SSR, somatostatin-receptors; VEGF, vascular endothelial growth factors; VEGFR, vascular endothelial growth receptors.

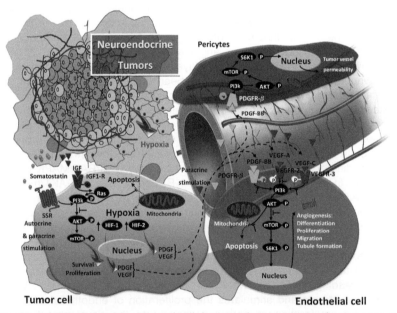

Fig. 2. Hypoxia-driven angiogenesis and cellular interplays in neuroendocrine tumors. HIF, hypoxia inducible factor; mTOR, mammalian target of rapamycin; PDGF, platelet derived growth factors; PDGFR, platelet derived growth receptors; SSR, somatostatin receptors; VEGF, vascular endothelial growth factors; VEGFR, vascular endothelial growth receptors.

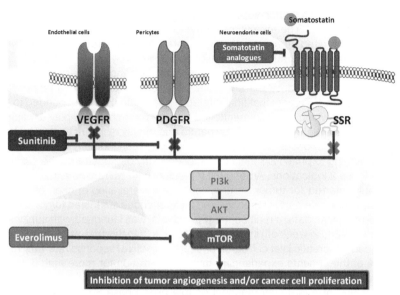

Fig. 3. Mechanisms of action of targeted drugs in neuroendocrine tumors. mTOR, mammalian target of rapamycin; PDGFR, platelet derived growth receptors; SSR, somatostatin receptors; VEGFR, vascular endothelial growth receptors.

derived from rapamycin such as everolimus specifically bind to mTOR and may block signal transduction in tumor cells as well as in cells involved in tumor angiogenesis.

INHIBITION OF VEGFR AND PDGFR BY SUNITINIB IN NETS

Angiogenesis has been shown to play a crucial role in the development of NETs in humans.[9] For instance, PNETs have a well-developed vasculature and are VEGF driven, suggesting a possible role for angiogenesis inhibitors in their treatment.[33,34] Well-differentiated NETs seem to express higher levels of HIF-1α, VEGF, and microvessel density than poorly differentiated NETs, suggesting the important role of tumor angiogenesis in the maintenance of NETs.[9] Although data remain limited, it seems that higher levels of angiogenesis can be observed in tumors with a low level of cancer cell proliferation, as measured by Ki67 expression. Furthermore, immunohistochemical analysis of tissue from malignant PNETs also shows widespread expression of PDGFR-α and PDGFR-β, stem cell factor receptor (c-KIT), VEGFR-2 and VEGFR-3, and epidermal growth factor receptors.[9,33,34] Considering that VEGFR plays a major role in endothelial cell survival and that PDGFR plays a similar function in pericytes, both VEGFR and PDGFR seem to be interesting potential targets for therapeutic interventions in well-differentiated NETs.

Sunitinib, an antiangiogenic agent approved for the treatment of advanced renal cell carcinoma and imatinib-resistant or intolerant gastrointestinal stromal tumors (GISTs), inhibits VEGFR-1, VEGFR-2 and VEGFR-3; PDGFR-α and PDGFR-β; and KIT, in addition to FMS-like tyrosine kinase 3, colony-stimulating factor-1 receptor (CSF-1R), and glial cell line–derived neurotrophic factor receptor (rearranged during transfection; RET), providing rationale for evaluation of sunitinib in NETs.[37,38] Furthermore, data on sunitinib in the RIP1-Tag2 transgenic mouse model of pancreatic islet cell tumors demonstrated a 75% reduction in the density of endothelial cells and a 63% reduction in pericyte coverage of tumor vessels as a result of the inhibition of VEGFR and PDGFR, respectively.[39] The magnitude of the effect was greater than when VEGFR or PDGFR was inhibited alone, suggesting a potential for greater therapeutic benefit when both of the receptor families are inhibited concurrently.[40]

During the course of the phase 1 trial with sunitinib, the authors witnessed strong anti-tumor activity as reflected by the unusually high number of objective responses in several tumor types.[41] Tumors that first entered in phase 1 trials and responded to sunitinib were those in which the aforementioned kinases were shown to play a major role and those that were highly angiogenic by nature and mostly resistant to classical cytotoxic agents. First responses were observed in renal cell carcinoma and imatinib-resistant GISTs, leading to phase 2/3 trials that subsequently demonstrated the efficacy of sunitinib in those 2 indications. Among the 3 patients with NETs who entered phase 1 trials primarily referred for tumor progression after several lines of chemotherapy, 1 exhibited an impressive partial response and 2 experienced sustained tumor stabilizations. Based on these data, a multicenter phase 2 trial was launched with sunitinib (50 mg/d 4-week on and 2-week off) in patients with NETs.[42] In this trial, among 66 patients with advanced pancreatic islet cell carcinoma, the objective response rate was 16.7%, with 56.1% of the patients experiencing tumor stabilization for more than 6 months, leading to a median time to tumor progression of 7.7 months. This result set the basis for the launching of a large international double-blind phase 3 trial comparing 37.5 mg sunitinib (continuous dosing) with placebo in patients with well-differentiated PNETs progressing within 12 months before the study entry. Results from this trial showed a median progression-free survival of 11.1 months in patients treated with sunitinib as compared with 5.5 months in patients treated with placebo (HR, 0.397; $P<.001$).[43] The magnitude of benefit in this trial seems to be independent of the bulk of the liver involvement by the tumor, previous treatments, prior or concurrent use of somatostatin analogues, and the rate of expression of Ki67. Importantly, a survival improvement in patients treated with sunitinib was also observed in this trial. Adverse events were similar to those observed in other sunitinib studies and mainly consisted of neutropenia, hypertension, diarrhea, and hand-foot syndrome. Results from this study suggest that sunitinib has substantial antitumor activity with a good safety profile in patients with pancreatic islet cell tumors. Based on these data, approvals from the US Food and Drug Administration and European Medicines Agency have been requested for sunitinib in advanced PNET. It is likely that sunitinib, demonstrating efficacy in pancreatic islet cell carcinomas, will pave the way of further trials in other NET types, such as carcinoids, more poorly differentiated neuroendocrine diseases, and several other endocrine tumors that depend on VEGF/VEGFR for angiogenesis. Furthermore, based on these data, combinations of sunitinib with somatostatin analogues or chemotherapy may further be evaluated in upcoming clinical trials. Finally, this trial sets up the magnitude of benefit in terms of progression-free survival, which shall be expected from other targeted therapies currently investigated in PNET.

OTHER DRUGS TARGETING VEGF-DEPENDENT ANGIOGENESIS

Bevacizumab is a monoclonal antibody directed against VEGF. Bevacizumab is used in combination with various therapies in patients with advanced colon, breast, lung, and renal cell carcinomas. Considering the important role of VEGF in the growth of NETs,[44] bevacizumab was tested in a phase 2 trial in 44 patients with advanced or metastatic NETs randomly assigned to receive either bevacizumab (15 mg/kg every 3 weeks) or pegylated IFN-α2b.[45] Among 22 patients, 4 (18%) experienced partial response in the bevacizumab group compared with 0% in the IFN-α2b group.

Considering that only 40% patients had documented tumor progression at study entry, at 18 weeks, 96% of the patients treated with bevacizumab remained free of disease progression compared with 68% of patients treated with IFN-α2b. Grade 3 or 4 hypertension was present in 53% but was easily controlled with antihypertensive medications. Bevacizumab has demonstrated synergistic activities with several anticancer agents and a safe toxicity profile when combined with chemotherapy in numerous tumor types. As such, combinations of bevacizumab with streptozotocin, doxorubicin, and/or 5-fluorouracil or its derived oral mimetic capecitabine have attracted clinical interests and are currently proposed or tested in phase 2 clinical trials.

EVEROLIMUS AS A PARADIGM FOR mTOR inhibition

Several preclinical data consistently support the important role of the PI3k/AKT/mTOR signaling pathway in NET.[46,47] This pathway may be stimulated by upstream activation of VEGF/VEGFR, PDGF/PDGFR, and IGF/IGFR, which are considered as important tyrosine kinase growth factors and receptors in NET. The PI3k/AKT/mTOR pathway has long been considered as a major target for therapeutic intervention in cancer.[48,49] The PI3k/AKT/mTOR signaling pathway is under control of 2 tumor suppressor genes, TSC2 and PTEN, that usually repress cellular proliferation.[50,51] Chromosome arm 16p containing TSC2 has been found to be deleted in 37% of PNETs.[52,53] Furthermore, PTEN function (acting as a phosphatase reversing the effects of PI3k) has been found lacking in 10% to 29% of NETs.[54] Lower cytoplasmic staining of either PTEN or TSC2 correlated with tumor aggressiveness, functional status, proliferation index, presence of liver metastasis at diagnosis or follow-up, and time to progression in a recent study.[55] Furthermore, TSC2 staining correlated with disease-free and overall survival in patients with complete tumor resection. However, neither PTEN nor TSC2 were independent prognostic predictors in multivariate analysis. Several other evidences also support the involvement of the Akt/mTOR pathway in PNET tumorigenesis and progression. It has been shown that losses of TSC2 or PTEN expression reduce the inhibition of mTOR activity caused by hypoxia. Akt/mTOR is also involved in the growth and apoptosis of pancreatic islet cells. Furthermore, PTEN mutations or downregulation as well as Akt activation yielded the overexpression of cyclin D1, which negatively regulates TSC1-TSC2 function.[56] The lack of TSC2 expression may induce impaired PI3k/Akt activation by reducing PDGFRor insulin receptor substrate level, limiting tumorigenic potential.

Several rapamycin derivatives (eg, rapalogues) demonstrated antiproliferative effects in vitro and in vivo in cancer cells that lost PTEN expression. In vitro studies performed in PNET cell lines showed inhibition of proliferation and G0/G1 cell cycle arrest on exposure to rapamycin, temsirolimus, and everolimus.[57,58] As previously reported in several tumor models, exposure to rapalogues induced Akt activation in NET carcinoma cells, which is considered as a common molecular mechanism of resistance to mTOR inhibitors. So far, 2 clinical trials have evaluated the efficacy of mTOR inhibitors in PNET using either temsirolimus or everolimus.

Temsirolimus showed antitumor activity in phase 1 clinical trials.[59] In a phase 2 trial, 36 patients with documented progression of disease (21 with carcinoid tumors and 15 with islet cell tumors) were treated with 25 mg intravenous weekly doses of temsirolimus, with an overall response rate of 5.6%.[60]

Everolimus, a rapamycin derivative with activity in phase 1, was also investigated in NET trials.[61,62] Another open-label, phase 2 nonrandomized study (RAD001 In Advanced Neuroendocrine Tumors [RADIANT]-1) assessed the clinical activity of everolimus, 10 mg/d, in patients with metastatic PNETs who experienced progression on or after chemotherapy. In this study, patients were stratified according to prior octreotide therapy to receive everolimus (stratum one, 115 patients) or everolimus plus long-lasting octreotide (stratum two, 45 patients). In stratum one, 11 partial responses (9.6%), 78 stable diseases (67.8%), and a median progression-free survival of 9.7 months were observed. In stratum two, there were 2 partial responses (4.4%), 36 stable diseases (80%), and a median progression-free survival of 16.7 months. Coadministration of octreotide and everolimus did not affect exposure to either drug. Most adverse events were mild to moderate and were consistent with those previously seen when everolimus was used as a single agent. Based on these promising data, 2 large randomized trials have been initiated, the results of which are awaited. In RADIAN-2, 429 patients with low- and intermediate-grade NETs will be randomized to receive long-lasting octreotide with or without everolimus. In RADIAN-3, a total of 420 patients with advanced PNET will receive either everolimus or best supportive care with placebo. The results of everolimus in PNET were first reported at the 12th World Congress on gastrointestinal cancer. In RADIAN-3, 410 patients with advanced low or intermediate grade PNET and disease progression within 12 months were randomized from August 2007 to May 2009 to receive everolimus at the dose of 10 mg/d or placebo. PFS was the primary endpoint of this trial. Prior local and systemic therapies such as chemotherapy were allowed and given in about 50% of patients as well as the use of concurrent somatostatin analogs that were also prescribed to half of the patient population. The study allowed cross-over for patient treated with placebo at the time of tumor progression. Preliminary reports showed that about 34% of patients had >3 metastatic sites. Well and moderately differentiated PNET were registered in 17% and 15% of patients treated with sunitinib and placebo, respectively. The median PFS was 11.0 and 4.6 months in the everolimus and placebo groups, respectively (HR: 0.35, $P<.0001$). Despite PFS improvement, no benefit in overall survival was detectable in patients treated with everolimus. Although generally well tolerated, grade 3-4stomatitis and diarrhoeas were reported in 5% and 3% of patients, respectively. Considering that everolimus had activity in tumors that became resistant to sunitinib, the effects of this agent in patients progressing under sunitinib therapy may be studied in future clinical trials.

OTHER TARGETS FOR SYSTEMIC THERAPIES

Numerous potential targets are currently tested, including most serine/threonine kinases related downstream to receptor tyrosine kinases involved in the proliferation of NET cells. NETs frequently express both IGFs and their receptors (IGFRs) and, as such, potentially depend on autocrine stimulation by this pathway for growth and survival. In carcinoid tumor cell lines, exogenous IGF activates mTOR and increases cellular proliferation. Studies in NET cell lines showed apoptosis when cultured with the IGF inhibitor NVP-AEW541.[63] Several IGF inhibitors have been tested in clinical trials in several tumor types, yielding disappointing results. However, a phase 2 trial of an anti-IGFR monoclonal antibody MK0646 is ongoing for the treatment of carcinoid and islet cell tumors.

OTHER ANTICANCER AGENTS IN CLINICAL DEVELOPMENT
Temozolomide

Dacarbazine and its related oral derivative temozolomide are methylating agents that showed activity in some patients with NETs.[64,65] As for many other anticancer agents, activity of these drugs has been reported in small uncontrolled phase 2 trials, limiting the appraisal of clinical benefit in patients with NET.[66,67] These drugs display a more pronounced activity in pancreatic islet cell tumors than in carcinoid tumors. In an *Eastern Cooperative Oncology Group (*ECOG) phase 2 study of dacarbazine, 14 of the 42 patients (33%) with islet cell pancreatic carcinoma were reported to experience partial or complete responses. A Southwest Oncology Group study reported a response rate of 16% in 9 of 56 patients with metastatic carcinoid tumors receiving dacarbazine as a single agent. In a larger phase 2/3 ECOG trial, 250 patients were given dacarbazine after progression on streptozoto-cin-based therapy, with a modest overall response rate of 8%, leading to some confusion on the efficacy of this agent in NETs. Furthermore, toxicity was a major issue in both studies.

In a more recent phase 2 study, Kulke and colleagues[68] have evaluated the combi-nation of temozolomide and thalidomide in 29 patients with metastatic NETs. Patients received temozolomide at a dose of 150 mg/m^2 for 7 days every 2 weeks, with daily thalidomide at doses ranging from 50 to 400 mg. The overall response rate was close to 25%, including a 45% response rate in patients with PNETs and a 7% response rate in patients with carcinoids. However, several patients discontinued therapy because of treatment-related toxicity, including severe thalidomide-induced neuropathy and temozolomide-related lymphopenia with opportunistic infections.[69]

Kulke and colleagues[70] also retrospectively assessed 76 patients, 30 patients who received treatment with temozolomide and thalidomide from the above-mentioned study and 46 patients treated with a combination of temozolomide and bevacizumab. Response as defined by the *Response Evaluation Criteria In Solid Tumors* was seen in 11 of 35 patients (33%) with PNETs but in none of 38 patients with carcinoid tumors. In 21 available specimens, complete absence of O-6-methylguanine DNA methyltrans-ferase (MGMT) expression seemed to define patients with PNETs who achieved signif-icant benefit from temozolomide (5 of 8 PNETs and none of 13 carcinoid tumors), which indicated that the success of treatment with temozolomide might depend on the absence of MGMT expression.[71,72]

Overall, despite some encouraging evidences, the clinical benefit of temozolomide (and dacarbazine) in NETs remains to be demonstrated using prospective randomized trials in more stringently defined populations of patients with NETs. Furthermore, those trials may benefit from evaluating MGMT expression as a surrogate marker of activity in future temozolomide-based chemotherapy.[73]

DESIGN OF FUTURE CLINICAL TRIALS

Lessons learned from recent clinical trials suggest the importance of addressing the activity of novel anticancer agents using appropriate modern methodologies as used in other tumor types. Retrospective experiences from the companionate use of novel drugs are usually subject to methodological flaws that often lead to the over-estimation of the antitumor activity of most anticancer agents.[74] Prospective phase 2 trials may be preferred, using progression-free survival as a primary end point of activity rather than tumor response that often only partially reflected the efficacy of novel anticancer agents. Although clinically relevant, patient-related clinical outcome and control of symptoms may be regarded as a secondary end point of efficacy, at least until activity is demonstrated based on improved progression-free and survival parameters. Data from small phase 2 uncontrolled studies are usually insufficient to draw definitive conclusions on the efficacy of novel anticancer agents; they should be evaluated in properly designed randomized clinical trials. Patient characteristics as defined by inclusion criteria are crucial parameters for the interpretation of results from randomized trials, considering the large variability of disease outcomes. It seems that patients with clearly demonstrated tumor progression before randomization should be entered in prospective trials to avoid confusions in evaluating the antitumor effects of novel anticancer drugs with the natural history of slowly progressing NETs. Although NETs are rare tumors, results from large randomized trials pledge for cooperative efforts in designing multicenter international trials that were shown to be easy to complete within a reasonable time frame of an average of 2 years.

SUMMARY

Somatostatin analogues and sunitinib demonstrated antitumor activity in patients with NETs. Whereas somatostatin analogues showed activity in patients with carcinoid tumors and limited hepatic involvement, sunitinib demonstrated significant benefits for patients with PNETs. Results are awaited with everolimus alone and in combination with octreotide in patients with carcinoid tumors and PNETs. Novel strategies may now be designed using these anticancer agents to optimize the current treatment of patients with NETs.

REFERENCES

1. Halfdanarson TR, Rabe KG, Rubin J, et al. Pancreatic neuroendocrine tumors (PNETs): incidence, prognosis and recent trend toward improved survival. Ann Oncol 2008;19:1727–33.
2. Pape UF, Bohmig M, Berndt U, et al. Survival and clinical outcome of patients with neuroendocrine tumors of the gastroenteropancreatic tract in a German referral center. Ann N Y Acad Sci 2004;1014:222–33.
3. Arnold R. Endocrine tumours of the gastrointestinal tract. Introduction: definition, historical aspects, classification, staging, prognosis and therapeutic options. Best Pract Res Clin Gastroenterol 2005;19:491–505.
4. Klöppel G, Anlauf M. Epidemiology, tumour biology and histopathological classi-fication of neuroendocrine tumours of the gastrointestinal tract. Best Pract Res Clin Gastroenterol 2005;19:507–17.
5. Couvelard A, Deschamps L, Ravaud P, et al. Heterogeneity of tumor prognostic markers: a reproducibility study applied to liver metastases of pancreatic endo-crine tumors. Mod Pathol 2009;22:273–81.
6. Couvelard A, Scoazec JY. A TNM classification for digestive endocrine tumors of midgut and hindgut: proposals from the European Neuroendocrine Tumor Society (ENETS). Ann Pathol 2007;27:426–32.
7. Couvelard A, Hu J, Steers G, et al. Identification of potential therapeutic targets by gene-expression profiling in pancreatic endocrine tumors. Gastroenterology 2006;131:1597–610.
8. Rindi G, Klöppel G, Alhman H, et al. TNM staging of foregut (neuro)endocrine tumors: a consensus proposal including a grading system. Virchows Arch 2006; 449:395–401.
9. Couvelard A, O'Toole D, Turley H, et al. Microvascular density and hypoxia-induc-ible factor pathway in pancreatic endocrine tumours: negative correlation of microvascular density and VEGF expression with tumour progression. Br J Cancer 2005;17(92):94–101.
10. Ballian N, Loeffler AG, Rajamanickam V, et al. A simplified prognostic system for resected pancreatic neuroendocrine neoplasms. HPB (Oxford) 2009;11:422–8.
11. Moertel CG, Kvols LK, O'Connell MJ, et al. Treatment of neuroendocrine carcinomas with combined etoposide and cisplatin. Evidence of major

therapeutic activity in the anaplastic variants of these neoplasms. Cancer 1991;68:227–32.

12. Eriksson B, Annibale B, Bajetta E, et al. ENETS Consensus Guidelines for the Standards of Care in Neuroendocrine Tumors: chemotherapy in patients with neuroendocrine tumors. Neuroendocrinology 2009;90:214–9.

13. Yao KA, Talamonti MS, Nemcek A, et al. Indications and results of liver resection and hepatic chemoembolization for metastatic gastrointestinal neuroendocrine tumors. Surgery 2001;130:677–82.

14. Knigge U, Hansen CP, Stadil F. Interventional treatment of neuroendocrine liver metastases. Surgeon 2008;6:232–9.

15. Vilar E, Salazar R, Pérez-García J, et al. Chemotherapy and role of the proliferation marker Ki-67 in digestive neuroendocrine tumors. Endocr Relat Cancer 2007;14: 221–32.

16. Moertel CG, Hanley JA, Johnson LA. Streptozocin alone compared with streptozocin plus fluorouracil in the treatment of advanced islet-cell carcinoma. N Engl J Med 1980;303:1189–94.

17. Moertel CG, Lefkopoulo M, Lipsitz S, et al. Streptozocin-doxorubicin, streptozocin-fluorouracil or chlorozotocin in the treatment of advanced islet-cell carcinoma. N Engl J Med 1992;326:519–23.

18. Kouvaraki MA, Ajani JA, Hoff P, et al. Fluorouracil, doxorubicin, and streptozocin in the treatment of patients with locally advanced and metastatic pancreatic endocrine carcinomas. J Clin Oncol 2004;22:4762–71.

19. Heng PN, Saltz LB. Failure to confirm major objective antitumor activity for streptozocin and doxorubicin in the treatment of patients with advanced islet cell carcinoma. Cancer 1999;86:944–8.

20. McCollum AD, Kulke MH, Ryan DP, et al. Lack of efficacy of streptozocin and doxorubicin in patients with advanced pancreatic endocrine tumors. Am J Clin Oncol 2004;27:485–8.

21. Kumar U, Grant M. Somatostatin and somatostatin receptors. Results Probl Cell Differ 2010;50:137–84.

22. Modlin IM, Pavel M, Kidd M, et al. Review article: somatostatin analogs in the treatment of gastro-entero-pancreatic neuroendocrine (carcinoid) tumors. Aliment Pharmacol Ther 2010;31:169–88.

23. Oberg K, Kvols L, Caplin M, et al. Consensus report on the use of somatostatin analogs for the management of neuroendocrine tumors of the gastroentero-pancreatic system. Ann Oncol 2004;15:966–73.

24. Msaouel P, Galanis E, Koutsilieris M. Somatostatin and somatostatin receptors: implications for neoplastic growth and cancer biology. Expert Opin Investig Drugs 2009;18:1297–316.

25. Rinke A, Muller HH, Schade-Brittinger C, et al. Placebo-controlled, double-blind, prospective, randomized study on the effect of octreotide LAR in the control of tumor growth in patients with metastatic neuroendocrine midgut tumors: a report from the PROMID Study Group. J Clin Oncol 2009;27:4656–63.

26. Fazio N, de Braud F, Delle Fave G, et al. Interferon-alpha and somatostatin analog in patients with gastroenteropancreatic neuroendocrine carcinoma: single agent or combination? Ann Oncol 2007;18:13–9.

27. Kwekkeboom DJ, Teunissen JJ, Bakker WH, et al. Radiolabeled somatostatin analog [177Lu-DOTA0,Tyr3]octreotate in patients with endocrine gastroentero-pancreatic tumors. J Clin Oncol 2005;23:2754–62.

28. Valkema R, Pauwels S, Kvols LK, et al. Survival and response after peptide receptor radionuclide therapy with [90Y-DOTA0,Tyr3]octreotide in patients with

advanced gastroenteropancreatic neuroendocrine tumors. Semin Nucl Med 2006;36:147–56.

29. Waldherr C, Pless M, Maecke HR, et al. The clinical value of [90Y-DOTA]-D-Phe1-Tyr3-octreotide (90Y-DOTATOC) in the treatment of neuroendocrine tumours: a clinical phase II study. Ann Oncol 2001;12:941–5.

30. Waldherr C, Pless M, Maecke HR, et al. Tumor response and clinical benefit in neuroendocrine tumors after 7.4 GBq (90)Y-DOTATOC. J Nucl Med 2002;43:610–6.

31. Virgolini I, Britton K, Buscombe J, et al. In- and Y-DOTA-lanreotide: results and implications of the MAURITIUS trial. Semin Nucl Med 2002;32:148–55.

32. Kwekkeboom DJ, de Herder WW, Kam BL, et al. Treatment with the radiolabeled somatostatin analog [177 Lu-DOTA0,Tyr3] octreotate: toxicity, efficacy, and survival. J Clin Oncol 2008;26:2124–30.

33. Casanovas O, Hicklin DJ, Bergers G, et al. Drug resistance by evasion of antiangiogenic targeting of VEGF signaling in late-stage pancreatic islet tumors. Cancer Cell 2005;8:299–309.

34. Inoue M, Hager JH, Ferrara N, et al. VEGF-A has a critical, nonredundant role in angiogenic switching and pancreatic beta cell carcinogenesis. Cancer Cell 2002;1:193–202.

35. Fjallskog ML, Lejonklou MH, Oberg KE, et al. Expression of molecular targets for tyrosine kinase receptor antagonists in malignant endocrine pancreatic tumors. Clin Cancer Res 2003;9:1469–73.

36. Fjallskog ML, Hessman O, Eriksson B, et al. Upregulated expression of PDGF receptor beta in endocrine pancreatic tumors and metastases compared to normal endocrine pancreas. Acta Oncol 2007;46:741–6.

37. Faivre S, Demetri G, Sargent W, et al. Molecular basis for sunitinib efficacy and future clinical development. Nat Rev Drug Discov 2007;6:734–45.

38. Mendel DB, Laird AD, Xin X, et al. In vivo antitumor activity of SU11248, a novel tyrosine kinase inhibitor targeting vascular endothelial growth factor and platelet-derived growth factor receptors: determination of a pharmacokinetic/pharmaco-dynamic relationship. Clin Cancer Res 2003;9:327–37.

39. Pietras K, Hanahan D. A multitargeted, metronomic, and maximum-tolerated dose "chemo-switch" regimen is antiangiogenic, producing objective responses and survival benefit in a mouse model of cancer. J Clin Oncol 2005;23:939–52.

40. Yao VJ, Sennino B, Davis RB, et al. Combined anti-VEGFR and anti-PDGFR actions of sunitinib on blood vessels in preclinical tumor models. In: Programs and abstract of the 18th EORTC-NCI-AACR Symposium on Molecular Targets and Cancer Therapeutics. Prague: 2006 0 AD/11/7.

41. Faivre S, Delbaldo C, Vera K, et al. Safety, pharmacokinetic, and antitumor activity of SU11248, a novel oral multitarget tyrosine kinase inhibitor, in patients with cancer. J Clin Oncol 2006;24:25–35.

42. Kulke MH, Lenz HJ, Meropol NJ, et al. Activity of sunitinib in patients with advanced neuroendocrine tumors. J Clin Oncol 2008;26:3403–10.

43. Raymond E, Faivre S, Hammel P, et al. Sunitinib paves the way for targeted therapies in neuroendocrine tumors. Target Oncol 2009;4:253–4.

44. Zhang J, Jia Z, Li Q, et al. Elevated expression of vascular endothelial growth factor correlates with increased angiogenesis and decreased progression-free survival among patients with low-grade neuroendocrine tumors. Cancer 2007;109:1478–86.

45. Yao JC, Phan A, Hoff PM, et al. Targeting vascular endothelial growth factor in advanced carcinoid tumor: a random assignment phase II study of depot octreotide with bevacizumab and pegylated interferon alpha-2b. J Clin Oncol 2008;26:1316–23.

46. Missiaglia E, Dalai I, Barbi S, et al. Pancreatic endocrine tumors: expression profiling evidences a role for AKT-mTOR pathway. J Clin Oncol 2010;28: 245–55.
47. Capdevila J, Salazar R. Molecular targeted therapies in the treatment of gastro-enteropancreatic neuroendocrine tumors. Target Oncol 2009;4:287–96.
48. Faivre S, Kroemer G, Raymond E. Current development of mTOR inhibitors as anticancer agents. Nat Rev Drug Discov 2006;5:671–88.
49. Vignot S, Faivre S, Aguirre D, et al. mTOR-targeted therapy of cancer with rapamycin derivatives. Ann Oncol 2005;16:525–37.
50. Zhang H, Cicchetti G, Onda H, et al. Loss of Tsc1/Tsc2 activates mTOR and disrupts PI3K-Akt signaling through downregulation of PDGFR. J Clin Invest 2003;112:1223–33.
51. Zhang H, Bajraszewski N, Wu E, et al. PDGFRs are critical for PI3K/Akt activation and negatively regulated by mTOR. J Clin Invest 2007;117:730–8.
52. Chung DC, Brown SB, Graeme-Cook F, et al. Localization of putative tumor suppressor loci by genome-wide allelotyping in human pancreatic endocrine tumors. Cancer Res 1998;58:3706–11.
53. Rigaud G, Missiaglia E, Moore PS, et al. High resolution allelotype of nonfunctional pancreatic endocrine tumors: Identification of two molecular subgroups with clinical implications. Cancer Res 2001;61:285–92.
54. Perren A, Komminoth P, Saremaslani P, et al. Mutation and expression analyses reveal differential subcellular compartmentalization of PTEN in endocrine pancreatic tumors compared to normal islet cells. Am J Pathol 2000;157: 1097–103.
55. Kaper F, Dornhoefer N, Giaccia A. Mutations in the PI3K/PTEN/TSC2 pathway contribute to mammalian target of rapamycin activity and increased translation under hypoxic conditions. Cancer Res 2006;66:1561–9.
56. Guo SS, Wu X, Shimoide AT, et al. Frequent overexpression of cyclin D1 in sporadic pancreatic endocrine tumours. J Endocrinol 2003;179:73–9.
57. Grozinsky-Glasberg S, Franchi G, Teng M, et al. Octreotide and the mTOR inhibitor RAD001 (everolimus) block proliferation and interact with the Akt-mTOR-p70S6K pathway in a neuro-endocrine tumour cell line. Neuroendocrinology 2008;87:168–81.
58. Zitzmann K, De Toni EN, Brand S, et al. The novel mTOR inhibitor RAD001 (everolimus) induces antiproliferative effects in human pancreatic neuroendocrine tumor cells. Neuroendocrinology 2007;85:54–60.
59. Raymond E, Alexandre J, Faivre S, et al. Safety and pharmacokinetics of escalated doses of weekly intravenous infusion of CCI-779, a novel mTOR inhibitor, in patients with cancer. J Clin Oncol 2004;22:2336–47.
60. Duran I, Kortmansky J, Singh D, et al. A phase II clinical and pharmacodynamic study of temsirolimus in advanced neuroendocrine carcinomas. Br J Cancer 2006;95:1148–54.
61. O'Donnell A, Faivre S, Burris HA 3rd, et al. Phase I pharmacokinetic and pharmacodynamic study of the oral mammalian target of rapamycin inhibitor everolimus in patients with advanced solid tumors. J Clin Oncol 2008;26:1588–95.
62. Yao JC, Phan AT, Chang DZ, et al. Efficacy of RAD001 (everolimus) and octreotide LAR in advanced low- to intermediate-grade neuroendocrine tumors: Results of a phase II study. J Clin Oncol 2008;26:4311–8.
63. Höpfner M, Baradari V, Huether A, et al. The insulin-like growth factor receptor 1 is a promising target for novel treatment approaches in neuroendocrine gastrointestinal tumours. Endocr Relat Cancer 2006;13:135–49.

64. Strosberg JR, Kvols LK. A review of the current clinical trials for gastroentero-pancreatic neuroendocrine tumours. Expert Opin Investig Drugs 2007;16: 219–24.

65. Arnold R, Rinke A, Schmidt CH, et al. Endocrine tumours of the gastrointestinal tract: Chemotherapy. Best Pract Res Clin Gastroenterol 2005;19:649–56.

66. Ekeblad S, Sundin A, Janson ET, et al. Temozolomide as monotherapy is effective in treatment of advanced malignant neuroendocrine tumors. Clin Cancer Res 2007;13:2986–91.

67. Maire F, Hammel P, Faivre S, et al. Temozolomide: a safe and effective treatment for malignant digestive endocrine tumors. Neuroendocrinology 2009;90:67–72.

68. Kulke MH, Stuart K, Enzinger PC, et al. Phase II study of temozolomide and thalidomide in patients with metastatic neuroendocrine tumors. J Clin Oncol 2006;24:401–6.

69. Schwarzberg AB, Stover EH, Sengupta T, et al. Selective lymphopenia and opportunistic infections in neuroendocrine tumor patients receiving temozolomide. Cancer Invest 2007;25:249–55.

70. Kulke MH, Frauenhoffer S, Hooshmand SM, et al. Prediction of response to temozolomide (TMZ)-based therapy by loss of MGMT expression in patients with advanced neuroendocrine tumors (NET) [abstract 4505]. In programs and abstracts of the 2007 ASCO Annual Meeting. Chicago (IL), June 1–5, 2007. p. S18.

71. Bracht LK, Wen P, Meyerhardt JA, et al. DNA repair enzyme expression and differential response to temozolomide in a patient with both glioblastoma and metastatic pancreatic neuroendocrine tumor. J Clin Oncol 2008;26:4843–4.

72. Kulke MH, Hornick JL, Frauenhoffer C, et al. O6-methylguanine DNA methyltransferase deficiency and response to temozolomide-based therapy in patients with neuroendocrine tumors. Clin Cancer Res 2009;15:338–45.

73. Gounaris I, Rahamim J, Shivasankar S, et al. Marked response to a cisplatin/docetaxel/temozolomide combination in a heavily pretreated patient with metastatic large cell neuroendocrine lung carcinoma. Anticancer Drugs 2007;18:1227–30.

74. Eriksson B. New drugs in neuroendocrine tumors: rising of new therapeutic philosophies? Curr Opin Oncol 2010;22:381–6.

Nutrition and Gastroenteropancreatic Neuroendocrine Tumors

Vay Liang W. Go, MD[a],*, Priya Srihari[b],
Leigh Anne Kamerman Burns, MS, LDN, RD[c]

KEYWORDS

- Diet • Nutrition • Metabolism • Neuroendocrine tumors

Gastroenteropancreatic (GEP) neuroendocrine tumors (NETs) are relatively rare neoplasms that characteristically synthesize and secrete an excess of a variety of regulatory peptides, hormones, and neuroamines, which regulate gut and pancreatic function. This excess can lead to distinct clinical syndromes.[1,2] However, some GEP NETs are clinically silent until there are mass effects in their presentation with metastases. Therapeutic strategies include surgery, radiofrequency ablation, chemotherapy, chemoembolization, and biotherapy using somatostatin analogs.[3,4] The clinical syndromes and the various management strategies can lead to altered gut and pancreatic function with nutritional consequences. Nutritional and dietary management is critical for GEP NET patients and is the focus of this article.

NEUROENDOCRINE REGULATION OF GUT-NUTRITION-METABOLISM AXIS

The gastrointestinal system plays an integral role in the assimilation of all nutrients from the diet. The macronutrients (carbohydrates, fats, and proteins) undergo digestion in the intestinal lumen by secreted enzymes from the pancreas and gut and in the brush-border surface for the intestinal mucosa. This is followed by absorption by enterocytes and subsequent transport of digestive products through the circulation. This entire process is highly regulated by the neuroendocrine system, including the autonomic nervous system, numerous gastrointestinal hormones, and regulatory

This work was supported by Grant No. AT003960 NCCAM from the National Institutes of Health.

The authors have nothing to disclose.

[a] UCLA Center for Excellence in Pancreatic Diseases, David Geffen School of Medicine at UCLA, 900 Veteran Avenue, Warren Hall 13-146, Los Angeles, CA 90095–1786, USA

[b] UCLA Center for Excellence in Pancreatic Diseases, David Geffen School of Medicine at UCLA, 900 Veteran Avenue, Warren Hall 13-146, Los Angeles, CA 90095–1786, USA

[c] Cancer Prevention Liaisons, LSUHSC School of Medicine New Orleans, Stanley S. Scott Cancer Center, 533 Bolivar Street, New Orleans, LA 70112–1249, USA

* Corresponding author.

E-mail address: vlwgo@ucla.edu

peptides, which act as paracrine, autocrine, and neurocrine pathways. Ingested food and absorbed nutrients provide well-coordinated gut functions including secretion, digestion, motility, and absorption.[5]

Neurohormonal regulation of gastric and pancreatic exocrine and endocrine secretion after a meal can be classified into the cephalic, gastric, and intestinal phases. The cephalic phase is initiated by sight, smell, taste, chewing, and swallowing of food and is mediated in the brainstem, posterior nucleus tractus solitarius, dorsal motor nucleus, and cortical nervous system. This phase activates vagal efferent impulses that stimulate both gastric and pancreatic secretion. The gastric phase occurs when food and fluids are present in the gastric lumen. Fifty percent of total acid secretion is stimulated by the meal. The greater the gastric distention, the greater is this acid secretion. The vagal nerve fibers mediate this phase and also regulate gastrin secretion. The intestinal phase is initiated by the entry of gastric chyme into the duodenum and the upper intestine. Quantitatively, this phase accounts for less than 10% of gastric acid secretion, but more importantly it regulates most of the pancreatic exocrine and endocrine secretion. This phase is primarily mediated by activating cholinergic reflexes and the release of gastrointestinal hormones, such as cholecystokinin (CCK), secretin, gastric inhibitory polypeptide, and glucagon-like peptide-1. These various hormones do regulate pancreatic endocrine secretions, insulin, glucagon, somatostatin, pancreatic polypeptide, and the secretion of digestive enzymes from the exocrine pancreas.

The various regions of the small intestine perform key digestive and absorptive functions. The duodenum and jejunum are the major sites of digestion and absorption of carbohydrates, proteins, and fats, and of absorption of most vitamins and minerals. Fat-soluble vitamins are integrated into the process of dietary lipid absorption, whereas water-soluble vitamins typically have their own mechanism for transport across the intestinal membrane. The ileum is the major site for absorption of water, electrolytes, and bile acids. The colon is the principal site of absorption of electrolytes and water. In addition, colonic bacteria provide the main source of short-chain fatty acids, such as acetate and butyrate. The transit of gastric and intestinal chymes is well coordinated by gastrointestinal motility, also under neurohormonal regulation.

The role of nutrients in the neurohormonal regulation of food intake and metabolism has been well documented (**Fig. 1**). Evidence now exists that nutrients have acquired a mechanistic and regulatory function in addition to the traditional concept of constituents of diet that serve as a significant energy-yielding substrate and as a precursor for the synthesis of macromolecules or components in normal cell differentiation, growth, renewal, and repair.[5,6] Nutrients could influence and regulate gene transcription, translation, and posttranslational metabolic processes. Moreover, they could regulate the release of gut neuroendocrine peptides that regulate motor, secretory, and absorptive functions, and the release of the metabolic hormone insulin. The neuropeptides released, such as CCK, could then act in both the circulation and vagal neural pathways, and interact with leptin peripherally in addition to its central action in regulate of satiety. In addition, leptin, being a long-term adiposity signal, may also increase the efficacy of CCK through interactions initiated at peripheral gastrointestinal sites or at dual sites with central leptin sensitizing the PVN to respond to inputs generated by the short-term satiety factor, CCK. The role of other gut neuropeptides on the peripheral actions of the neural vagal-sympathetic fibers need to be further investigated.

It is well established that neurohormonal pathways in the brain, gut, and adipose tissues play a key role in nutrient metabolism and fuel homeostasis, and it is also now established that nutrients (ie, glucose, free fatty acids, and amino acids) can

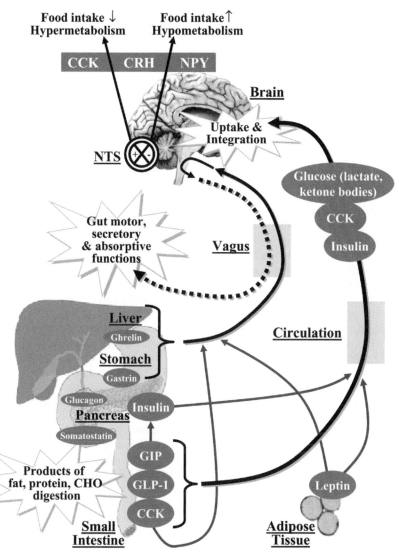

Fig. 1. The role of nutrients in the regulation of gut neuroendocrine system that activate vagal afferent fiber, interact with leptin synergistically to reduce food intake, and influence vagal efferent pathway to regulate gut motor, secretory, and absorptive functions. CCK, cholecystokinin; CHO, carbohydrate; CRH, corticotrophin-releasing hormone; GIP, gastrointestinal inhibitory peptide; GLP-1, glucagon-like peptide 1; NPY, neuropeptide Y; NTS, nucleus tract solitaries. (*Modified from* Go VLW, Wang Y, Yang H, et al. Neuro-hormonal integration of metabolism: challenges and opportunities in the postgenomic era. In: Allison SP, Go VLW, editors. Metabolic issues of clinical nutrition. Nestle Nutrition Workshop Series Clinical and Performance Program. Vevey/S. Kanger A.G. Basil 2004;9:227–42; with permission.)

regulate and modulate neurohormonal factors that affect metabolism at the cellular, organ-system, and whole-body levels. In this postgenomic era with genomic technology, this complex multiple nutrient metabolism and its control regulatory system can be analyzed simultaneously, from gene expression to metabolic flux to metabolic phenotype affecting cell cycles and growth, development, and apoptosis, to quality of life and the dietary requirements of the individual.

NETS AFFECT GUT FUNCTION-METABOLISM

Most NETs are small (<1 cm) and slow growing (months to years). They usually metastasize to the liver and bone before becoming symptomatic, often when the tumor is larger than 2 cm. NETs may have episodic expression and may be silent for years. They are often misdiagnosed, because their symptoms complex mimics other common disorders. Most GEP NETs are carcinoid tumors followed by insulinoma, pancreatic polypeptide, gastrinoma, VIPoma, glucagonoma, somatostatinoma, ghrelinoma, multiple endocrine neoplasia type I and type II, and other rare tumors.[3] Because of their rarity, for the most part endocrinologists make their living not by diagnosing and treating NETs, but rather by excluding disorders that masquerade as NETs. Perturbation of the gut's nutrition-metabolism process occurs in GEP NETs because of their excessive production of gastrointestinal hormones, peptides, and amines, which can lead to maldigestion, diarrhea, steatorrhea, and altered gastrointestinal motility that develops into various clinical syndromes (**Table 1**).[3] Gastrinoma, Zollinger-Ellison syndrome, is characterized by gastric hyperacidity caused by gastrin hypersecretion from islet cell tumors or the duodenum. Approximately 90% of gastrinomas are found in the "gastrinoma triangle," an area bordered by the confluence of the cystic and common ducts superiorly, the lateral sweep of the "C" loop of the duodenum, and the mesenteric vessels medially. The classic description of insulinoma is the Whipple triad, whose symptoms complex includes hypoglycemia with low blood glucose relieved by ingestion of glucose. Most insulinomas are benign and can be located anywhere within the pancreas. In contrast, ghrelinoma, caused by excessive production of ghrelin, a gastric hormone, can cause hyperglycemia, insulin deficiency or resistance, and intestinal dysmotility. Glucagonoma is characterized by skin rash, dermatosis, deep venous thrombosis, depression, and diarrhea. Somatostatinoma is caused by hypersecretion of somatostatin. The salient features of this tumor include diarrhea and steatorrhea; diabetes; cholelithiasis; and dysmotility and hypochlorhydria caused by the inhibitory effect of somatostatin on gastrointestinal secretion, motility, and gut and pancreatic hormone secretion. In some GEP NETs, multiple hormones or peptides are responsible for symptoms or multiple tumors involving several organs, such as in multiple endocrine neoplasia type I and type II, and can confound the clinical diagnosis of NETs. Any surgical approaches that remove or alter the anatomy of the gastrointestinal tract or biotherapy, such as the need for somatostatin analogs that suppress the secretion of gastrointestinal pancreatic hormones and function, can also lead to alteration of gastrointestinal secretory, motor, and absorptive functions. The tumor production of an excess of a variety of regulatory peptides, the surgical management, or biotherapy with synthetic somatostatin analogs could have both dietary and nutritional consequences.

DIETARY MANAGEMENT IN PATIENTS WITH NETS

Because of the intricacy of the NET symptom complex before, during, and after patient therapy and the specific nutritional needs related to the course of NETs, a registered dietician should be part of the multidisciplinary health care team. Unfortunately, there are a limited number of registered dieticians and physicians who have expertise in the nutritional management of NETs. Currently, there are also no national dietary guidelines developed specifically for NETs. The pioneering work of Warner's "Nutritional Concerns for the Carcinoid Patient" in 2000 has led her to develop nutritional guidelines for the carcinoid patient, available at the Carcinoid Cancer Foundation.[7] These guidelines were updated in 2009. This is one of the key resources related to the field. The objectives of nutrition management are to assist in the development of individualized nutrition care plans, to promote optimal nutritional status, and to evaluate the effectiveness of nutritional approaches, with an overall goal to improve the quality of life of the patient during therapy. The best diet for an NET patient largely depends on whether or not the patient is symptomatic, the stage of the disease, and the type of therapeutic management.

For patients with newly diagnosed NETs without symptoms, it is prudent to follow the healthy diet based on the Dietary Guidelines for Americans, 2005, for health promotion and chronic disease prevention including cancer (**Box 1**).[8] The United States Dietary Guidelines for Americans is the latest scientific evidence-based review in nutrition, and provides information and advice for choosing a nutritious diet, maintaining a healthy weight, achieving adequate exercise, and keeping foods safe to avoid food-borne illness. The recommendations are translated for implementation by the US Department of Agriculture Food Guidance in My Pyramid, which has been continuously updated (**Fig. 2**) with the DASH Eating Plan.[9,10] These recommendation guidelines are similar to those suggested by the American Cancer Society, World Health Organization, and other academic societies and institutes of medicine, including the American Institute for Cancer Research, which has published *The New American Plate Cookbook*, containing recipes for a healthy weight and a healthy life.[11] The healthy diet is primarily a plant-based diet, with 5 to 10 servings of fruits and vegetables and less animal protein, substituting beans and other legumes for protein instead. It also consists of low-fat or fat-free dairy; foods with a good source of healthy fats, such as nuts and seeds, which are low in saturated fat and contain no trans fatty acids; and whole grains as a source of carbohydrates. This diet also limits salt and refined sugar intake. Dietary supplements should also be avoided unless recommended by a physician. The 2005 Dietary Guidelines for Americans is currently being updated by the Department of Health and the US Department of Agriculture Advisory Committee for the 2010 Dietary Guidelines. Unfortunately, their anticipated report has not yet been released.[12]

Most GEP NET patients are cancer survivors, primarily because of the advancement of various therapeutic and diagnostic procedures. The quality of life related to dietary guidelines has received major interest. In recent studies conducted by the American Cancer Society, there have been three major recommendations for all cancer survivors regarding lifestyle: 150 minutes of moderate or strenuous physical activity or 60 minutes of strenuous activity per week, at least five servings of fruits and vegetables per day, and no smoking.[13] This study indicated that less than 5% of the surveyed survivors meet all three recommendations, but those who did observed a better health-related quality of life. Population-based studies have shown that approximately 48% to 74% are not meeting the recommended five servings a day of fruits and vegetables, whereas this particular study revealed that 80% to 85.2% of survivors were not meeting the five-a-day recommendation. Although there was a higher correlation with physical activity and better health-related quality of life, previous research has shown that in survivors of some cancers, eating five servings of fruits and vegetables is negatively associated with depression, which in turn is negatively associated with health-related quality of life. The Neuroendocrine Unit at the Eastern Virginia Medical School examined quality of life in a more exclusive group of patients with NETs. They developed the Norfolk Quality of Life Tool, a questionnaire of 72 questions that determined the domains that had a great impact on NET patient quality of life.[14] The resulting data were separated into the domains of physical functioning, respiratory, depression,

Table 1
The clinical presentations, syndromes, tumor types, sites, and hormones

Clinical Presentation	Syndrome	Tumor Type	Sites	Hormones
Flushing	Carcinoid	Carcinoid	Gastric, mid, and foregut, pancreas/ foregut, adrenal medulla	Serotonin, substance P, NKA, TCT, PP, CGRP, VIP
Diarrhea	Carcinoid WDHHA ZE MCT PP	Carcinoid VIPoma Gastrinoma Medullary carcinoma PPoma	As above Pancreas, mast cells Pancreas, duodenum Thyroid, pancreas Pancreas	As above VIP Gastrin Calcitonin PP
Diarrhea/Steatorrhea	Somatostatin	Somatostatinoma, neurofibromatosis	Pancreas, duodenum, bleeding gastrointestinal tract	Somatostatin
Wheezing	Carcinoid	Carcinoid	Gut/pancreas, lung	Serotonin, substance P, chromogranin A
Dyspepsia, ulcer disease, low pH on endoscopy	ZE	Gastrinoma	Pancreas (85%), duodenum (15%)	Gastrin
Hypoglycemia	Whippier triad	Insulinoma Sarcomas Hepatoma	Pancreas Retroperitoneal Liver	Insulin IGF/binding protein IGF
Dermatitis	Sweet syndrome Pellagra	Glucagonoma Carcinoid	Pancreas Midgut	Glucagon Serotonin
Dementia	Sweet syndrome	Glucagonoma	Pancreas	Glucagon

Clinical feature	Syndrome	Tumor	Location	Mediator
Diabetes	Glucagonoma	Glucagonoma	Pancreas	Glucagon
	Somatostatin	Somatostatinoma	Pancreas	Somatostatin
Deep venous thrombosis	Somatostatin	Somatostatinoma	Pancreas	Somatostatin
Steatorrhea	Somatostatin	Somatostatinoma	Pancreas	Somatostatin
Cholelithiasis/ neurofibromatosis	Somatostatin	Somatostatinoma	Pancreas	Somatostatin
Silent/liver metastases	PPoma	PPoma	Pancreas	PP
Acromegaly/ gigantism	Acromegaly	Neuroendocrine tumors	Pancreas	GH-RH
Cushing disease	Cushing	Neuroendocrine tumors	Pancreas	ACTH/CRF
Anorexia, nausea, vomiting	Hypercalcemia	Neuroendocrine tumors	Pancreas	PTHRP
Constipation, abdominal pain		VIPoma	Pancreas	VIP
Pigmentation		Neuroendocrine tumors	Pancreas	VIP
Postgastrectomy	Dumping, syncope, tachycardia, hypotension, borborygmus, explosive diarrhea, diaphoresis, mental confusion	None	Stomach/duodenum	Osmolarity, insulin, GLP

Abbreviations: ACTH, adrenocorticotropic hormone; CGRP, calcitonin gene-related peptide; CRF, corticotropin-releasing factor; GH-RH, growth hormone–releasing hormone; GLP, glucagon-like peptide; IGF, insulin-like growth factor; MCT, medullary carcinoma of thyroid; NKA, neurokinin A; PP, pancreatic polypeptide; PTHRP, parathyroid hormone receptor; TCT, thyrocalcitonin; VIP, vasoactive intestinal polypeptide; WDHHA, watery diarrhea syndrome; ZE, Zollinger-Ellison syndrome.

Data from Mamikuniam G, Vinik AI, O'Dorisio TM, Woltering EA, Go VLW. Neuroendocrine tumors, a comprehensive guide to diagnoses and management. 4th edition. California: Interscience Institute; 2009.

Box 1
Recommendations by the 2005 Dietary Guidelines Advisory Committee

- Monitor your body weight to achieve health
- Be physically active each day
- Choose a variety of foods with, and among, the basic food groups, while not exceeding your daily calorie limit
- Increase daily intake of fruits and vegetables, whole grains, and non-fat or low-fat milk and milk products
- Keep food safe to eat
- Decrease intake of saturated fat, trans fat, and cholesterol while increasing foods rich in omega-3 fatty acids (fish)
- Choose and prepare foods with less salt
- If you drink alcoholic beverages, do so in moderation

From US Department of Health and Human Services, US Department of Agriculture. Dietary guidelines for Americans 2005. Washington: US Government Printing Office; 2005.

---

cardiovascular, gastrointestinal, flushing, and positive or negative attitude. The questionnaire results further demonstrated that four particular domains were significant in NET patients: (1) physical functioning, (2) flushing, (3) gastrointestinal effects, and (4) depression. The nutrition and diet of patients can impact these domains.

Regarding the nutritional considerations for symptomatic NETs patients, it is advisable to follow the healthy diet plan recommended for nonsymptomatic patients, as described previously. However, every individual must weigh general advice against their own experience and symptoms complex. The most common symptoms complex includes diarrhea, abdominal pain, gas and bloating, and flushing. Lesser symptoms include fatigue, weakness, weight loss, and skin rash. There are some key nutritional

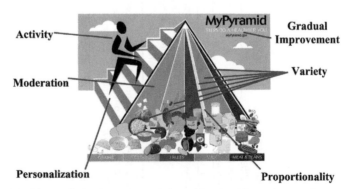

Anatomy of MyPyramid
One Size Doesn't Fit All

Fig. 2. Modified figure from the USDA Web-based food guidance system. (*From* MyPyramid. gov. US Department of Agriculture. Available at: http://www.mypyramid.gov/index.html. Updated March 24, 2010. Accessed April 27, 2010.)

issues to consider for this group of patients. They should avoid high amine-containing foods (**Box 2**). Avoiding spicy foods and alcoholic beverages may also help to prevent flushing.

There are several dietary substitutions that patients with NETs have learned can help their diarrhea. These include ripe bananas, pureed vegetables, and cooked or canned fruits, such as applesauce, instead of raw vegetables in the form of salad, fresh or dried fruit, pickles, and relishes. Rice, pasta, and potatoes can be substituted in place of high-fiber vegetables, such as cabbage. Other substitutions include jam or jelly on whole grain bread instead of cream cheese or butter on white bread; clear broth soup instead of creamy soup; crackers or pretzels in place of doughnuts and butter cookies; electrolyte replacements drinks, such as Gatorade, instead of carbonated soft drinks or fruit juice with pulp; and lactose-free beverages and products instead of regular milk and dairy products. It is important to determine whether the diarrhea is caused by the underlying endocrine tumors, such as VIPoma, gastrinoma, or carcinoid tumors, rather than other secretory diarrhea related to bacterial toxins, such as those in food poisoning, lactose intolerance, medications containing laxatives, or part of an irritable bowel syndrome. Loperamide or opiates have also been used for symptomatic improvement of NET-related diarrhea.

Currently, two somatostatin analogs, octreotide and lanreotide, are used to control symptoms of patients with NETs. Recently a multi-institutional German research group reported their results that the octreotide LAR significantly improves the time to progression among patients with metastatic, well-differentiated midgut NETs.[15] Their results also suggested the stabilizing effect of somatostatin analogs in NETs. Both synthetic somatostatin analogs are highly selective for somatostatin 2 receptors and have a prolonged plasma half-life with respect to somatostatin. Use of these

---

Box 2
Amine-rich foods and products (tyramine, dopamine)

High

- Aged cheeses (cheddar, Camembert, Stilton)
- Alcoholic beverages
- Smoked, salted, or picked fish or meat (herring, salami, sausage, corned beef, bologna, pepperoni)
- Any spoiled protein foods (chicken liver)
- Yeast extracts and brewer's yeast, hydrolyzed proteins
- Broad beans, sauerkraut, shrimp paste, some soybean products, miso soup, soy sauce, tofu

Moderately high

- Caffeine-containing drinks, coffee (in large amounts), soda
- Chocolate (in large amounts)
- Some nuts (peanuts, coconuts, Brazil nuts)
- Some pizzas, raspberries, banana, avocado

Data from Warner M. Nutritional concerns for the carcinoid patient: developing nutrition guidelines for persons with carcinoid disease. Carcinoid Cancer Foundation Web site. Available at: http://carcinoid.org/pcf/lectures/docs/MwarnerlectureSept2.htm. Updated 2009. Accessed April 6, 2010.

analogs, which have all the biologic action of somatostatin in suppression of the gastrointestinal tract and pancreatic function, can lead to fat maldigestion and altered fat and fat-soluble vitamin absorption.[16] The adverse effects of somatostatin analog therapy are similar to those observed in somatostatinoma patients, which include steatorrhea, gas, nonspecific gastrointestinal discomfort, hyperglycemia, and hypo-thyroidism. Periodic monitoring of glucose metabolism, thyroid function, and plasma vitamins D and B_{12} levels is recommended.

Systemic chemotherapy and combination therapy with somatostatin analogs, inter-feron, mTOR inhibitors, or vascular endothelial growth factor inhibitors are currently used. These therapies do have additional side effects including anorexia, weight loss, and liver function abnormalities.[17,18] Nutritional assessment and dietary changes need to be monitored and coordinated with the health care team.

There are other nutritional considerations in NET management. (1) Niacin deficiency can occur as a result of increased tryptophan metabolism into serotonin. This could lead to dermatitis, diarrhea, dementia, and death caused by pellagra. A daily supple-ment of 25 to 50 mg should be taken. (2) Another consideration is that pancreatic enzymes, such as pancrease, creon, and ultrase, are recommended for patients with steatorrhea, particularly related to somatostatin analog therapy. (3) Fat-soluble vitamins A, D, E, and K, and multiple vitamins are also advisable, particularly if the patient has fat malabsorption. (4) Maintaining an ideal body weight and preventing weight loss is important in monitoring the nutritional status of the patient. (5) In post-surgery patients, any alteration of gut anatomy can lead to malabsorption. Dietary changes and an appropriate nutritional care plan should be specifically developed for particular individuals. (6) Nutraceuticals or dietary supplements are used with caution. They may interfere with various chemotherapies, and there is a lack of evidence-based data to support their use.

SUMMARY

Nutritional assessment and development of nutrition care plans are an integral part of the multidisciplinary management team for patients with NETs. Registered dietitians or physicians with expertise in nutrition can provide dietary approaches to improve the quality of life and nutritional status during various therapeutic modalities used in patients with NETs. They can monitor these patients and provide appropriate dietary changes to address the various side effects of therapy.

It is prudent to follow the Dietary Guidelines for Americans for health promotion and disease prevention including cancer. A prospective clinical trial focused on investi-gating nutritional status as a consequence of the course and various types of NETs is urgently needed to provide the appropriate database in the development of an evidence-based dietary guideline specifically for patients with NETs.

REFERENCES

1. Modlin IM, Oberg K, Chung DC, et al. Gastroenteropancreatic neuroendocrine tumors. Lancet Oncol 2008;9(1):61–72.
2. Vinik AI, Silva MP, Woltering G, et al. Biochemical testing for neuroendocrine tumors. Pancreas 2009;38(8):876–89.
3. Mamikuniam G, Vinik AI, O'Dorisio TM, et al. Neuroendocrine tumors, a compre-hensive guide to diagnoses and management. 4th edition. Los Angeles (CA): In-terscience Institute; 2009.
4. Plockinger U, Rindi G, Arnold R, et al. Guidelines for the diagnosis and treatment of neuroendocrine gastrointestinal tumors. A consensus statement on behalf of

the European Neuroendocrine Tumor Society (ENETS). Neuroendocrinology 2004;80:394–424.

5. Go VLW, Wang Y, Yang H, et al. Neuro-hormonal integration of metabolism: challenges and opportunities in the postgenomic era. In: Allison SP, Go VL, editors, Metabolic issues of clinical nutrition. Nestle Nutrition Workshop Series Clinical and Performance Program. Switzerland: Vevey/S. Kanger A.G. Basil; 2004:9. p. 227–42.

6. Go VLW, Wong DA, Wang Y, et al. Prevention: evidence-based medicine to genomic medicine. J Nutr 2004;134:3513S–6S.

7. Warner M. Nutritional concerns for the carcinoid patient: developing nutrition guidelines for persons with carcinoid disease. Carcinoid Cancer Foundation Web site. Available at: http://carcinoid.org/pcf/lectures/docs/MwarnerlectureSept2.htm. Updated 2009. Accessed April 6, 2010.

8. Dietary Guidelines for Americans 2005. Washington: US Government Printing Office: Dietary Guidelines Advisory Committee; US Department of Health and Human Services, US Department of Agriculture; 2005.

9. MyPyramid.gov. US Department of Agriculture. Available at: http://www.mypyramid.gov/index.html. Updated March 24, 2010. Accessed April 27, 2010.

10. Karanja NM, Obarzanek E, Lin P, et al. The DASH eating plan at 1,600-, 2,000-, 2,600-, and 3, 1000-calorie levels. J Am Dent Assoc 1999;8:S19–27.

11. American Institute for Cancer Research. The new American plate cookbook. Berkeley (CA): University of California Press; 2005.

12. Dietary Guidelines for Americans Web Site. Available at: http://www.health.gov/dietaryguidelines/. Updated October 8, 2009. Accessed May 5, 2010.

13. Blanchard CM, Courneya KS, Stein K. Cancer survivors' adherence to lifestyle behavior recommendations and associations with health-related quality of life: results from the American Cancer Society's SCS-II. J Clin Oncol 2008;26(13): 2198–204.

14. Vinik E, Carlton CA, Silva MP, et al. Development of the Norfolk Quality of Life Tool for assessing patients with neuroendocrine tumors. Pancreas 2009;38(3): e87–95.

15. Rinke A, Muller HH, Schade-Brittinger C, et al. Placebo-controlled, double-blind, prospective, randomized study on the effect of octreotide LAR in the control of tumor growth in patients with metastatic neuroendocrine midgut tumors: a report from the PROMID study group. J Clin Oncol 2009;27:4656–63.

16. Öberg K, Kaltsas G, Ferone D, et al. Standards of care in neuroendocrine tumors: biotherapy. Neuroendocrinology 2009;90(2):209–13.

17. Yao JC, Phan AT, Chang DZ, et al. Efficacy of RAD001 (everolimus) and octreotide LAR in advanced low-to-intermediate grade neuroendocrine tumors: results of a phase II study. J Clin Oncol 2008;26:4311–8.

18. Yao JC, Phan A, Hoff PM, et al. Targeting vascular endothelial growth factor in advanced carcinoid tumor: a random assignment phase II study of depot octreotide with bevacizumab and pegylated interferon alpha-2b. J Clin Oncol 2008;26: 1316–23.

The Role of Angiogenesis in Neuroendocrine Tumors

John Lyons III, MD, Catherine T. Anthony, PhD,
Eugene A. Woltering, MD*

KEYWORDS

- Angiogenesis • i-MTOR inhibitors
- Vascular endothelial growth factor (VEGF)
- Platelet-derived growth factor (PDGF)
- Human in vitro modeling • Somatostatin receptors

Angiogenesis is the process by which new capillaries develop from previously formed venules. Adult angiogenesis exists in a few normal (physiologic) settings, such as menstruation. Angiogenesis is rare in adults except in pathologic settings, such as rheumatoid arthritis. This size represents proliferative retinopathies, psoriasis, and tumor growth. Both benign and malignant tumors must develop their own blood supply to grow larger than 2 mm in size, the limits of effective simple diffusion of oxygen and nutrients and the removal of metabolic waste products.

The angiogenesis response is triggered by an "angiogenic switch" that occurs when the concentration or actions of proangiogenic agents exceeds those of antiangiogenic agents.[1] The concept of an angiogenic switch and its key role in the modulation of new blood vessel growth has led researchers to search for more than three decades for agents responsible for inducing and for inhibiting angiogenesis.

Somatostatin, or somatomedin release-inhibiting factor (SRIF), was originally described in 1968.[2] It is an endogenenous peptide known for its ubiquitous inhibitory capacity on gastrointestinal function. SRIF inhibits gastrointestinal motility, amine release, peptide release, growth factor synthesis and release, and the secretion of a variety of fluids. Although this inhibitory capacity was attractive to clinicians wishing to inhibit bowel fluid secretion and to decrease bowel motility, SRIF's short half-life limited the compound's clinical usefulness. The limited half-life of the native peptide led to the development of longer lasting, more potent analogs or congeners of somatostatin. These novel peptides have been used since the 1980s in a variety of clinical situations, including limiting the peptide hypersecretion from tumors of

Department of Surgery, Louisiana State University, Health Sciences Center, New Orleans, LA 70112, USA
* Corresponding author.
E-mail address: ewolte@lsuhsc.edu

Endocrinol Metab Clin N Am 39 (2010) 839–852
doi:10.1016/j.ecl.2010.08.006
0889-8529/10/$ – see front matter © 2010 Elsevier Inc. All rights reserved.

gastroenteropancreatic axis.[3] In the late 1980s, reports began to surface that somatostatin analogs could produce not only the relief of clinical symptoms due to amine or peptide excess but also an antitumor effect.[4] Some researchers hypothesized that this antitumor effect was the result of inhibition of angiogenesis. This seemed like a logical theory considering the nearly universal inhibitory abilities of these somatostatin analogs. Fassler and colleagues[5] were the first to test the antiangiogenic effects of octreotide. In 1988, they presented preliminary data supporting the antiangiogenic effects of octreotide acetate in a few chicken eggs using the chicken chorioallantoic membrane (CAM) model. These investigators demonstrated that octreotide acetate could inhibit blood vessel growth. This theory was further investigated by Woltering and colleagues[6] using the CAM. The CAM is an assay popularized by Dr Judah Folkman,[7] the father of the angiogenesis concept. In the CAM model, fertilized chick eggs are placed in a 37°C incubator. On day 2 or 3 of development, the embryos are removed from their shell and placed in a plastic wrap hammock and reincubated. On day 6 or 7, a methylcelluose disc containing a test substance is placed on the outer third of the CAM. The radius of the zone of inhibition of blood vessels is visually assessed 24 to 48 hours after disc implantation. Woltering and colleagues tested the angiogenic potential of both SMS 201-995 (octreotide) and RC-160 (vapreotide). Both somatostatin analogs inhibited angiogenesis, but RC-160 demonstrated a slightly higher percentage of eggs exhibiting inhibition of angiogenesis and a higher degree of overall growth inhibition. These effects were dose dependent. Another finding from these studies was that the degree of angiogenic inhibition was similar to that of the positive (inhibitory) control, a combination of heparin and a steroid, hydrocortisone 21-phosphate. The Folkman group used this steroid along with a heparin facilitator to inhibit capillary growth and had proposed this mixture as a potential chemotherapeutic.[8] The observation that Folkman's steroid required the presence of heparin to inhibit capillary growth,[9] whereas the somatostatin analogs inhibited angiogenesis without such a facilitator, suggested that the effect of somatostatin analogs may occur directly on the cell's membrane, acting through specific somatostatin receptors.

In an effort to better understand the ability of somatostatin to inhibit angiogenesis, Barrie and colleagues[10] compared the angiogenic potential of native somastatin-14 and eight novel somatostatin analogs in the CAM model. These investigators found that the inhibitory ability of these molecules varied greatly. This variation in potency depended on the structure of the analog and its specific amino acid sequence (**Fig. 1** and **Table 1**). This finding implied that certain analogs bound to specific somatostatin receptor subtypes (sst) with varying degrees of affinity. The most potent drugs in this study were cyclic octapeptides that retained a lysine in position 5 and a cysteine at positions 2 and 7 (forming a cysteine-cysteine bridge). The substitution of the position 5 lysine for ornithine, an amino acid not found in mammalian biosynthesis, rendered the analog biologically inactive. These data also suggested that a specific ligand/receptor interaction was required in order for somatostatin analogs to confer different biologic responses, including their antiangiogenic effects. Furthermore, these studies demonstrated that there was a direct correlation between an analog's effectiveness as antiangiogenic agent and its affinity for sst 2. Those analogs with better growth hormone inhibitory ability also bound to sst 2 with greater affinity and were more potent antiangiogenic agents.[11]

In an attempt to determine the specific signal transduction mechanisms responsible for somatostatin-induced angiogenic inhibition, Patel and colleagues[12] tested octreotide alone and in combination with blockers of specific postreceptor signal transduction pathways.[12] These investigators found that octreotide's inhibition of angiogenesis was G-protein dependent and adenylate cyclase dependent. Octreotide was also

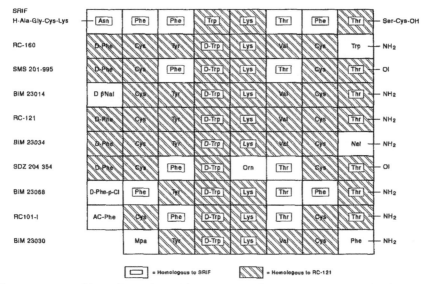

Fig. 1. Amino acid homology of peptide sequences of various somatostatin analogs with native somatostatin-14 (SRIF). (*From* Barrie R, Woltering EA, Hajarizadeh H, et al. Inhibition of angiogenesis by somatostatin and somatostatin-like compounds is structurally dependent. J Surg Res 1993;55(4):446; with permission.)

Table 1
Angiogenesis inhibition somatostatin analogs compared with native somatostatin-14

Test Substance	% Inhibition	RPR
SRIF	26	1
RC-160	68[a,b]	2.6
SMS 201-995	61[a,b]	2.3
BIM 23,014C	46[a,b]	1.8
RC 121	35	1.3
BIM 23,034[c]	25	1.0
SDZ 204-354	12	0.5
BIM 23,068	10	0.4
BIM 23,030	0	0
Pos. control	71	2.7
Lyoph buffer	14	0.5
Buffer	3	0–1

Relative potency ratios are the percentage of inhibition induced by an analogue divided by the percent inhibition of angiogenesis induced by native somatostatin. SMS 201–995 is octreotide acetate. The positive control is hydrocortisone 21-phosphate.

Abbreviations: Lyoph buffer, lypholysed buffer; NR, not reported; Pos. control, positive control; RPR, relative potency ratio; SRIF, somadomedin release inhibiting factor.

[a] Different from SRIF (P<.05).
[b] Different from buffer (P≤.05).
[c] Opaque disks.

Data from Woltering EA, Watson JC, Alperin-Lea RC, et al. Somatostatin analogs: angiogenesis inhibitors with novel mechanisms of action. Invest New Drugs 1997;15:77–86.

found to act along calcium-dependent pathways. Octreotide's angiogenic inhibitory potency was significantly decreased when this analog was combined with either bradykinin, an agent that drives calcium across the cell membrane, or extracellular hypercalcemia. Verapamil, an L-calcium channel blocker, was able to reverse the effects of bradykinin and hypercalcemia and to restore octreotide's ability to inhibit angiogenesis.

Unfortunately, the CAM model has significant limitations. The most obvious limitation of this model is that it uses animal, not human, tissues as its target. Additionally, the blood vessel response that is assessed in this growing chick embryo is more akin to vasculogenesis and embryogenesis than to true angiogenesis. To overcome the issue of embryogenesis, somatostatin analogs were tested against porcine endothelial cells and smooth muscle cells.[13] Octreotide inhibited cell proliferation of both cell types. Danesi and colleagues[14] demonstrated similar results using human umbilical vein endothelial cells (HUVECs). This group found that octreotide at 10^{-9} M reduced the proliferation of HUVECs by 45% versus untreated controls.

Some of the limitations of the CAM model were overcome with the development of a model that used full-thickness, 3-D, intact mammalian tissues. One of the first such models was a murine model of ex vivo angiogenesis developed by Nicosia and Ottinetti.[15] Briefly, thoracic aortas were harvested from Fischer 344 male rats, sectioned into rings of 1-mm length, and placed into either fibrin or collagen gels. The investigators found that the aortic rings generated branching microvessels using serum-free media in both fibrin and collagen gels. These microvessels were inhibited by the addition of hydrocortisone and upregulated with the addition of medium conditioned with sarcoma 180 cells.[15] Although this model overcame the issue of embryogenesis as was observed in the CAM, it was limited due to the use of animal tissues as its medium.

To counter the limitations imposed by animal-based cell or organ culture systems, Woltering and colleagues[16] developed a unique assay that uses human tissues embedded in a fibrin-thrombin clot as a source of proliferating neovessels. Human placental vein discs are harvested and used as targets in a fibrin-thrombin clot assay to evaluate angiogenesis. These veins normally possess monolayers of quiescent endothelial cells in their intima. When the full-thickness sheets of vein are cut into small discs with a 2-mm skin punch, the mechanical trauma to the vein creates injury and a stressful milieu at the vessel's cut edge. Such an environment is sufficient to turn on the angiogenic switch, stimulating these previously quiescent endothelial cells to begin to proliferate in a manner similar to that which occurs in wounding in vivo. Angiogenic neovessels then proliferate from the cut edge of the vein disc (**Fig. 2**). These neovessel sprouts assays have lumens, and they interconnect and have all of the attributes of human capillaries. Transmission electron microscopy has been used to confirm that placental vein neovessel sprouts are endothelial in nature as they exhibit both Weibel-Palade bodies and tight junctions (**Fig. 3**).[17] The endothelial nature of these sprouts has also been confirmed with immunohistochemical stains for factor VIII.[16] Briefly, 2-mm discs of placental vein are placed into the thrombin-loaded wells and covered with a clot-forming nutrient medium containing fibrinogen. This mixture is incubated at 37°C, allowing a fibrin-thrombin clot to form. Once a tissue-containing clot is formed, control wells are treated with nutrient medium containing fetal bovine serum whereas experimental wells are incubated in an identical nutrient medium plus the test reagent. Tissue-containing wells are examined under an inverted phase microscope after 14 days of incubation. A semiquantitative grading system developed and validated in the Woltering laboratory is used to visually assess the degree of neovascularization.

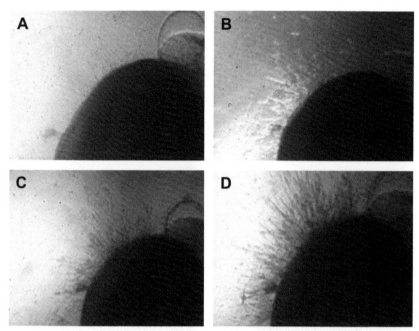

Fig. 2. Evaluation of angiogenesis. Tissue disks were divided into four quadrants with each quadrant given a numeric score from 0 to 4 based on neovessel length, density, and percentage of the quadrant's circumference involved with the angiogenic response. Numeric results from the four quadrants were summed and expressed as a semiquantative AI (AI, 0–16). Panels *A–D* depict tissue disks with quadrant AI values of 1–4, respectively. (*From* Stafford SJ, Schwimer J, Anthony CT, et al. Colchicine and 2-methoxyestradiol inhibit human angiogenesis. J Surg Res 2005;125(1):104–8; with permission.)

The knowledge that a somatostatin analog's antiangiogenic effectiveness is directly proportional to its sst 2–binding affinity[11] led Watson and colleagues[18] to hypothesize that proliferating human vascular endothelial cells express sst 2 whereas quiescent ones do not. To test this hypothesis, they used human tissues in the previously described fibrin-thrombin clot assay. They embedded placental vein discs from six anonymous donors into fibrin-thrombin clots and assessed their angiogenic response on day 15. Those discs that demonstrated endothelial cell growth from the cut edge of the disc were deemed to be proliferating and those viable discs that lacked endothelial cell growth were deemed to have remained quiescent. These investigators demonstrated for the first time that sst 2 gene expression was universally present in proliferating vascular endothelium but sst 2 expression was uniquely absent in quiescent endothelium derived from tissue-matched placental vein samples.

To confirm these reverse transcriptase–polymerase chain reaction (RT-PCR) results, immunohistochemical staining using anti–sst 2 antiserum was performed in proliferating and nonproliferating discs. These selective stains revealed that proliferating endothelium stained positive for sst 2 receptors whereas quiescent endothelium did not. These observations were extended into an animal model. Nude mice were implanted with neuroblastoma tumor cells that lacked the sst 2 receptor as measured by RT-PCR and in vitro assays. When the tumors were approximately 2 cm, mice were injected with ^{125}I-WOC4a, a radiolabeled, sst 2–preferring somatostatin analog. Nuclear medicine scans and radiographs were performed in register. Significant

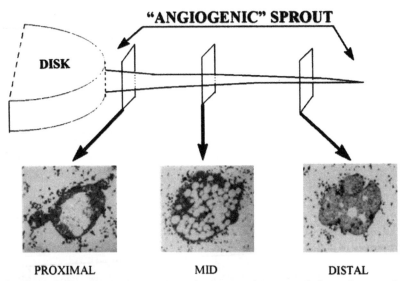

Fig. 3. Electron microscopic examination of microvessel outgrowth from the cut edge of a human placental vein disc. Capillary cross-sections: proximal (original magnification ×4200), mid (original magnification ×2000), and distal (original magnification ×2700). (*From* Watson JC, Redmann JG, Meyers MO, et al. Breast cancer increases initiation of angiogenesis without accelerating neovessel growth rate. Surgery 1997;122:509–14; with permission.)

uptake was observed in the tumor whereas non–tumor-bearing sites did not accumulate radioligand (except for the liver, which was the normal route of excretion for the radiolabeled peptide). The binding seen in the tumors was thought to be the result of sst 2 receptor expression on angiogenesis blood vessels supplying the tumor.

An additional advantage of the fibrin-thrombin clot assay is its ability to test human tumor specimens against a variety of antiangiogenic agents over a wide range of concentrations. Similar to the method used to plate vein discs, fresh human tumors harvested at operation can be made into 1-mm³ fragments and embedded in the fibrin-thrombin clots.[19] As neovessels sprout from the tumor's cut edge, the angiogenic response can then be quantified by the percent of specimens that begin to grow (percent initiation) or the degree of neovessel growth (angiogenic index [AI]) or the overall effect of the drug (overall drug effect). Unlike vein discs, which possess only resting endothelial cells, tumor fragments harbor actively proliferating endothelial cells in their existing angiogenic vessels. This tumor-based fibrin-thrombin clot assay was used to further investigate the presence of sst 2 receptors on angiogenic blood vessels.[20] Two different tumor types, one whose tumor cells were sst 2 positive and the other whose tumor cells were sst 2 negative, were implanted in the fibrin-thrombin clot assay. Both were allowed to develop an angiogenic response (presumably sst 2 positive). Then both tumor models were treated with an sst 2–favoring radiolabeled somatostatin analog. Tumoricidal effects were seen only in the sst 2–positive tumor cells, whereas antiangiogenic effects were seen in both tumor types. The investigators concluded that although sst 2s were present on the tumor cells of only one of the tumors, sst 2s were present on the neovessels of both tumors.

To date, many tumor types have been studied in this fibrin-thrombin clot assay. These include breast, colon, and ovarian cancers as well as malignant neuroendocrine tumors (NETs). Carcinoid tumors and islet cell tumors (ICTs) have been extensively studied in this assay using a wide variety of clinically available agents, such as taxol, vincristine, vinblastine, and octreotide acetate. In addition, a variety of experimental reagents that are still in clinical development have been used against these NET specimens, including 2-methoxyestradiol (2-MeOH), rapamycin, vatalanib (PTK787/ ZK222584), everolimus (RAD-001), and pasireotide (SOM-230), an sst 1-, 2-, 3-, and 5-preferring somatostatin analog.

Stafford and colleagues[21] used this fibrin-thrombin clot assay to study the antiangiogenic profile of tubulin inhibitors against human neovessels. Two tubulin inhibitors that were investigated were colchicine and 2-MeOH. Colchicine, an older drug used commonly in the treatment of gout, has been shown to inhibit tumor growth by triggering cell cycle arrest in the G2/M phase and by inducing apoptosis. A natural metabolite of 17-estradiol, 2-MeOH has been recently discovered to be far more potent than cholcicine.[22] It has also shown to maintain potent apoptotic activity against rapidly growing tumor cells and endothelial cells.[23,24] These investigators used placental vein discs from three separate human placentas and encouraged them to develop an angiogenic response in the fibrin-thrombin clot assay. Both colchicine and 2-MeOH were tested against these neovessels over a wide range of concentrations (10^{-6} to 10^{-12} M). The investigators observed that both colchicine and 2-MeOH exhibited antiangiogenic properties. The doses of colchicine required to induce antiangiogenesis, however, was much greater than the maximum tolerated human dose, negating its clinical use as an effective antiangiogenic agent. 2-MeOH inhibited neovessel growth and angiogenic initiation at 10^{-6} M. This inhibitory dose was consistent with the IC50 (2–5×10^{-6} M) observed by other investigators who have tested this drug in animal models.[25] Based on these data, Stafford and colleagues proposed that 2-MeOH should be tested as an antiangiogenic in human clinical trials.

Antiangiogenic properties of tubulin inhibitors were further studied in NETs using this assay. Woltering and colleagues[16] hypothesized the epothilone B (Epo), a naturally occurring macrolide that inhibits cell proliferation by stabilizing microtubules, would inhibit angiogenesis. They tested human tissues using two different assay methodologies. In the first set of experiments, eight tumors (including five carcinoids) and four normal tissues were treated with either nutrient medium or drug-containing medium starting on the first day in culture. This was designed to represent the effect of early or neoadjuvant Epo treatment on the development of a tumor- or normal tissue–derived angiogenic response. In a second set of experiments, three tumors (two carcinoids and a parathyroid adenoma) and three normal tissues were allowed to develop an angiogenic response for 14 to 18 days, and then they were treated with either control medium or drug-containing medium for 1 to 2 weeks. This method allowed tumors or normal tissues to develop an angiogenic response before treatment, and it was developed to more accurately determine the therapeutic response of developed, mature neovessel networks, such as those seen in widely metastatic tumors. Epo at drug levels of 10^{-8} M or greater inhibited angiogenesis in the majority of tissues studied. This antiangiogenic effect was seen in both sets of experiments (early and late drug application), and it was observed in carcinoid tumors as well, a group of NETs that are typically unresponsive to chemotherapy in vivo.[26] The effective drug levels of Epo were consistent with the range of blood levels seen when this drug was tested in phase 1 trials.

Most recently, experiments using this assay have extended into the investigation of the vascular endothelial growth factor (VEGF) pathway in human tissues. Lyons and colleagues[27] hypothesized that the addition of VEGF to the placental vein disc or human tumor specimen–containing wells would stimulate angiogenesis and while anti-VEGF regimens would inhibit angiogenesis. To test these hypotheses, discs of human placental veins (physiologic model) and fragments of human tumors (pathologic model) were embedded in fibrin-thrombin clots and treated with either VEGFA165 or anti-VEGF pathway reagents. The anti-VEGF drugs included bevacizumab, a humanized monoclonal antibody to VEGF; IMC-18F1 and IMC-1121, human monoclonal antibodies directed against VEGF R1 and VEGF R2, respectively; and vatalanib (PTK787/ZK222584; PTK/ZK), a tyrosine kinase inhibitor of all three primary VEGF receptors (VEGF R1, R2, and R3) and several non-VEGF receptors, such as platelet-derived growth factor receptor. VEGF was tested against the vein discs of five separate human placentas and the fragments of eight separate malignant tumors, four of which were carcinoids. To the investigators' surprise, VEGF did not consistently stimulate neovascularization in human, vein-containing wells or in malignant tumor fragments. These experiments were repeated testing placental veins and malignant tumors (including carcinoids) with anti-VEGF reagents. Antibodies targeting VEGF R1 and VEGF R2 did not inhibit neovascularization in human tissues. Bevacizumab, although not affecting placental veins or gynecologic tumors, moderately inhibited angiogenesis in a subset of NETS (carcinoid tumors). In contrast, PTK/ZK significantly inhibited angiogenesis in every tissue type tested at multiple different concentrations. The inhibitory capacity of each molecule was proportional to the number of downstream targets that it affected. Antibodies to VEGF R1 and VEGF R2 affected only one target and had no inhibitory ability. Bevacizumab, an antibody that targets the VEGF-A ligand, affects all the receptors influenced by VEGF-A. This molecule had a modest inhibitory affect, but one that was greater than the antibodies to VEGF R1 and VEGF R2. PTK/ZK directly targets three primary VEGF receptors (R1, R2, and R3) as well as PDGF receptors and other non-VEGF receptors. PTK/ZK's inhibitory capacity was profound across all tissues and tumor types. This led the investigators to conclude that simply stimulating or blocking the VEGF pathway alone does not consistently alter neovascularization in human tissues. Manipulation of human neovessels was more consistently achieved when multiple growth factor pathways were affected simultaneously.

The fibrin-thrombin clot angiogenesis assay has been used extensively to study carcinoid tumors and ICTs. The ability to harvest an individual patient's tumor and to visually assess the angiogenic response of that tumor to a variety of agents potentially offers clinicians several unique opportunities to gauge a tumors' responsiveness to specific agents or pathways. These assays have the potential to make statements about the aggressiveness of a tumor. These assays may also enable clinicians to screen a variety of potentially usefully medications and to design a customized drug regimen with the best antiangiogenic potential for that individual.

Methods to screen the effects of chemotherapeutic agents against tumor cells have been widely reported for several decades. These assays were first reported by Hamburger and Salmon,[28] who described their in vitro soft agar culture system in 1977. The ability of these assays to choose effective chemotherapeutic agents was clinically evaluated when Von Hoff and colleagues[29] compared the clinical responses of patients who received a single reagent that was either picked by a clinician or picked by the assay. Patients who received an assay-guided drug enjoyed a 25% response rate whereas those given a clinician-selected reagent experienced a 15% response rate.[29] In contrast to chemosensitivity assays, Kern and Weisenthal[30] described a chemoresistance assay that exposes tumor specimens to suprapharmacologic concentrations of reagents. They have shown that drugs failing to suppress tumor growth at these extreme concentrations are likely to clinically fail 90% of the time. None of these chemosensitivity or chemoresistance assays

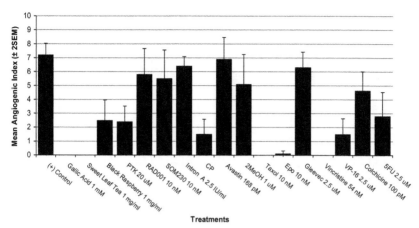

Fig. 4. One human carcinoid liver metastasis was tested against the 17 potential antiangiogenic drugs. Drugs with a lower angiogenic response are the better antiangiogenics in vitro. Avastin, bevacizumab; VP-16, etoposide; Gleevec, imantinib.

considers the blood vessel compartment of the tumor growth, however. The ability of fibrin-thrombin clot assay to assess the effect of therapy on neovessel growth makes this assay unique.

Figs. 4 and **5** outline the types of data that can be obtained from this fibrin-thrombin clot angiogenesis assay. **Fig. 4** illustrates data from one patient with a carcinoid. It outlines the angiogenic response in the fibrin-thrombin clot assay when tested with a panel of 17 different drugs. Drugs with a lower angiogenic response are the better antiangiogenics in vitro. Based on this data, it can be surmised that the most effective antiangiogenics in this carcinoid patient are gallic acid, sweet leaf tea, taxol, Epo, and vincristine, because they all significantly

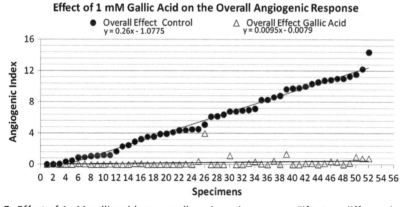

Fig. 5. Effect of 1mM gallic acid on overall angiogenic response. Fifty-two different human NETx were tested against the antiangiogenic drug, gallic acid. These different tumors are represented on the X axis as Specimens. Data were arranged in ascending order according to the control group's overall angiogenic response (0–16). Gallic acid consistently inhibited the overall angiogenic response, even in those specimens that had a robust control angiogenic response.

Table 2
Selected antiangiogenic agents tested in clinical trials

Agent	Carcinoid			Noncarcinoid NET		
	Complete Response	Partial Response	Stable Disease	Complete Response	Partial Response	Stable Disease
Bevacizumab + FOLFOX[34]	0/5 (0%)	1/5 (20%)	4/5 (80%)	0/7 (0%)	2/7 (29%)	5/9 (71%)
Bevacizumab + 2methoxyestradiol[35]	0/31 (0%)	0/31 (0%)	27/31 (93%)	NR	NR	NR
Bevacizumab + temozolamide[36]	0/12 (0%)	0/12 (0%)	11/12 (92%)	0/17 (0%)	4/17 (24%)	12/17 (70%)
Bevacizumab + Interferon[31]	0/22 (0%)	4/22 (18%)	17/22 (77%)	NR	NR	NR
Imantinib[37]	0/27 (0%)	1/27 (4%)	17/27 (63%)	NR	NR	NR
Imantinib[38]	0/2 (0%)	0/2 (0%)	1/2 (50%)	0/13 (0%)	0/13 (0%)	2/13 (15%)
Endostatin[39]	NR	NR	NR	0/40 (0%)[a]	0/40 (0%)[a]	32/40 (80%)[a]
Vatalanib[40]	NR	NR	NR	0/0 (0%)[a]	0/10 (0%)[a]	1/10 (10%)[a]
Atiprimod[41]	0/23 (0%)	0/23 (0%)	21/23 (91%)	NR	NR	NR
Gefitinib[42]	0/22 (0%)	0/22 (0%)	14/22 (64%)	0/15 (0%)	0/15 (0%)	2/15 (13%)
Sunitinib[33]	0/41 (0%)	1/41 (0%)	34/41 (83%)	0/66 (0%)	11/66 (17%)	45/66 (68%)
Sunitinib[32]	NR	NR	NR	2/86 (2%)	6/86 (7%)	NR
Sorafenib[43]	0/41 (0%)	4/41 (10%)	NR	0/41 (0%)	4/41 (10%)	NR
Everolimus + temozolamide[44]	NR	NR	NR	0/17 (0%)	6/17 (35%)	9/17 (53%)
Everolimus + octreotide[45]	0/30 (0%)	5/30 (17%)	24/30 (80%)	0/30 (0%)	8/30 (27%)	18/30 (60%)
Pasireotide[46]	0/11 (0%)	0/11 (0%)	9/11 (82%)	NR	NR	NR
Lanreotide[47]	NR	NR	NR	0/25 (0%)	1/25 (4%)	7/25 (28%)
Intron A[47]	NR	NR	NR	0/27 (0%)	1/27 (4%)	7/27 (26%)
Lanreotide + intron A[47]	NR	NR	NR	0/28 (0%)	2/28 (7%)	5/28 (18%)
Octreotide[48]	NR	NR	NR	0/42 (0%)[a]	1/42 (2%)[a]	28/42 (66%)[a]
5-fluorouracil + octreotide[49]	NR	NR	NR	0/29 (0%)	7/29 (24%)	20/29 (68%)
Thalidomide + temozolamide[50]	0/14 (0%)	1/14 (7%)	NR	1/14 (7%)	6/14 (43%)	19/28 (68%)[a]

Abbreviation: NR, not reported.
[a] This includes patients with carcinoid and noncarcinoid NETs because there was no clear distinction.

inhibited the overall angiogenic response. **Fig. 5** depicts the results of several patients (specimens 1–52) whose tumors were tested in vitro with the same antiangiogenic drug, gallic acid. In all 52 patients studied, gallic acid consistently inhibited neovascularization, even in those tumors with a robust control angiogenic response. Another notable point is that the specimen depicted in **Fig. 4** was harvested from a patient's liver metastasis. It has been occasionally observed that the same drug yields different antiangiogenic responses within the same patient depending on the harvest location of the specimen. In other words, a patient liver metastasis may significantly respond to gallic acid in vitro whereas his lymph node metastasis may not (data not shown). The potential for such intrapatient variability further underscores the importance of pretreatment drug screening.

Several investigators have tested antiangiogenic agents against carcinoids and other NETs in clinical trials. **Table 2** outlines selected clinical data that have been reported to date. Although complete responses to these reagents have been rare, many patients have experienced disease stabilization and some have enjoyed improved progression-free survival (PFS). Yao and colleagues[31] randomly assigned 44 patients with advanced carcinoid to receive 18 weeks of bevacizumab or pegylated interferon alfa-2b (intron A). Partial responses were observed in four (18%) patients receiving bevacizumab and zero (0%) receiving intron A. Stable and progressive disease was observed in 17 (77%) patients and 1 (5%) patient receiving bevacizumab, respectively, and 15 (68%) and 6 (27%) patients receiving intron A. The PFS rate after 18 weeks was 95% in the bevacizumab arm and 68% in the intron A the arm. Raymond and colleagues[32] evaluated another anti-VEGF reagent, sunitinib, versus placebo in patients with pancreatic ICTs. They also observed prolonged PFS in patients receiving antiangiogenic therapy (median PFS was 11 months after sunitinib vs 5 after placebo). Kulke and colleagues[33] evaluated this reagent in patients with both carcinoids and ICTs, and they found more objective tumor responses in patients with ICTs (16% vs 2%) than in patients with carcinoids. The median time to tumor progression was not significantly different between ICT patients and carcinoid patients (7 vs 10 months, respectively) nor was the 1-year survival rate (81% vs 83%, respectively).

The optimal drug regimen for patients with NETs has not yet been identified, but pretreatment in vitro drug screening to assess those drugs that are most likely to generate antiangiogenesis may hasten the ability to identify the most clinically efficacious drugs. Further investigations need to be made to clinically validate the angiogenic response observed with the fibrin-thrombin clot assay in vitro (ie, better understanding is needed of how a patient's in vitro response translates into a clinical outcome). Such information could enable avoiding futile medications in the future and customizing patients' therapy to drugs that are most likely to be affective against a NET.[31–50]

REFERENCES

1. Folkman J. Role of angiogenesis in tumor growth and metastasis. Semin Oncol 2002;29(6 Suppl 16):15–8.
2. Krulich L, Dhariwal AP, McCann SM. Stimulatory and inhibitory effects of purified hypothalamic extracts on growth hormone release from rat pituitary in vitro. Endocrinology 1968;83(4):783–90.
3. Pless J, Bauer W, Briner U, et al. Chemistry and pharmacology of SMS 201–995, a long-acting octapeptide analogue of somatostatin. Scand J Gastroenterol Suppl 1986;119:54–64.

4. Gorden P, Comi RJ, Maton PN, et al. NIH Conference. Somatostatin and somato-statin analogue (SMS 201–995) in treatment of hormone-secreting tumors of the pituitary and gastrointestinal tract and non-neoplastic diseases of the gut. Ann Intern Med 1989;110(1):35–50.

5. Fassler JA, O'Dorisio TM, Stevens RE, et al. Are somatostatin analogues anti-angiogenic? Clin Res 1988;36:869A.

6. Woltering EA, Barrie R, O'Dorisio TM, et al. Somatostatin analogues inhibit angio-genesis in the chick chorioallantoic membrane. J Surg Res 1991;50(3):245–51.

7. Folkman J. Proceedings: tumor angiogenesis factor. Cancer Res 1974;34(8): 2109–13.

8. Crum R, Szabo S, Folkman J. A new class of steroids inhibits angiogenesis in the presence of heparin or a heparin fragment. Science 1985;230(4732):1375–8.

9. Ingber DE, Madri JA, Folkman J. A possible mechanism for inhibition of angio-genesis by angiostatic steroids: induction of capillary basement membrane dissolution. Endocrinology 1986;119(4):1768–75.

10. Barrie R, Woltering EA, Hajarizadeh H, et al. Inhibition of angiogenesis by somatostatin and somatostatin-like compounds is structurally dependent. J Surg Res 1993;55(4):446–50.

11. Woltering EA, Watson JC, Alperin-Lea RC, et al. Somatostatin analogs: angiogenesis inhibitors with novel mechanisms of action. Invest New Drugs 1997;15(1):77–86.

12. Patel PC, Barrie R, Hill N, et al. Postreceptor signal transduction mechanisms involved in octreotide-induced inhibition of angiogenesis. Surgery 1994;116(6): 1148–52.

13. Sharma C, Alperin-Lea RC, Johnson MA, et al. Inhibition of octreotide acetate (o–a) on proliferation of porcine coronary artery smooth muscle, endothelium and fibroblasts cells [abstract]. FASEB J 1995;9(3).

14. Danesi R, Agen C, Benelli U, et al. Inhibition of experimental angiogenesis by the somatostatin analogue octreotide acetate (SMS 201–995). Clin Cancer Res 1997; 3(2):265–72.

15. Nicosia RF, Ottinetti A. Growth of microvessels in serum-free matrix culture of rat aorta. A quantitative assay of angiogenesis in vitro. Lab Invest 1990;63(1): 115–22.

16. Woltering EA, Lewis JM, Maxwell PJ 4th, et al. Development of a novel in vitro human tissue-based angiogenesis assay to evaluate the effect of antiangiogenic drugs. Ann Surg 2003;237(6):790–8 [discussion: 798–800].

17. Watson JC, Redmann JG, Meyers MO, et al. Breast cancer increases initiation of angiogenesis without accelerating neovessel growth rate. Surgery 1997;122: 509–14.

18. Watson JC, Balster DA, Gebhardt BM, et al. Growing vascular endothelial cells express somatostatin subtype 2 receptors. Br J Cancer 2001;85(2):266–72.

19. Gulec SA, Woltering EA. A new in vitro assay for human tumor angiogenesis: three-dimensional human tumor angiogenesis assay. Ann Surg Oncol 2004; 11(1):99–104.

20. Gulec SA, Drouant GJ, Fuselier J, et al. Antitumor and antiangiogenic effects of somatostatin receptor-targeted in situ radiation with 111In-DTPA-JIC 2DL. J Surg Res 2001;97(2):131–7.

21. Stafford SJ, Schwimer J, Anthony CT, et al. Colchicine and 2-methoxyestradiol inhibit human angiogenesis. J Surg Res 2005;125(1):104–8.

22. LaValee TM, Zhan XH, Herbstritt CJ, et al. 2-Methoxyestradiol inhibits proliferation and induces apoptosis independently of estrogen receptors a and b. Cancer Res 2002;62(13):3691–7.

23. Seegers JC, Lottering ML, Grobler CJS, et al. The mammalian metabolite 2-me-thoxyestradiol affects p53 levels and apoptosis induction in transformed cells but not normal cells. J Steroid Biochem Mol Biol 1997;62(4):253–67.

24. Fotsis T, Zhang Y, Pepper MS, et al. The endogenous oestrogen metabolite 2-me-thoxyestradiol inhibits angiogenesis and suppresses tumor growth. Nature 1994; 368(6468):237–9.

25. Schumacher G, Kataoka M, Roth JA, et al. Potent antitumor activity of 2-methox-yestradiol in human pancreatic cancer cell lines. Clin Cancer Res 1999;5(3): 493–9.

26. Kvols LK, Reubi JC. Metastatic carcinoid tumors and the malignant carcinoid syndrome. Acta Oncol 1993;32:197–201.

27. Lyons JM 3rd, Schwimer JE, Anthony CT, et al. The role of VEGF pathways in human physiologic and pathologic angiogenesis. J Surg Res 2010;159(1): 517–27.

28. Hamburger AW, Salmon SE. Primary bioassay of human tumor stem cells. Science 1977;197(4302):461–3.

29. Von Hoff DD, Clark GM, Stogdill BJ, et al. Prospective clinical trial of a human tumor cloning system. Cancer Res 1983;43:1926–31.

30. Kern DH, Weisenthal LM. Highly specific prediction of antineoplastic drug resis-tance with an in vitro assay using suprapharmacologic drug exposures. J Natl Cancer Inst 1990;82:582.

31. Yao JC, Phan A, Hoff PM, et al. Targeting vascular endothelial growth factor in advanced carcinoid tumor: a random assignment phase II study of depot octreo-tide with bevacizumab and pegylated interferon alpha-2b. J Clin Oncol 2008; 26(8):1316–23.

32. Raymond E, Niccoli-Sire P, Bang Y, et al. Updated results of the phase III trial of sunitinib (SU) versus placebo (PBO) for treatment of advanced pancreatic neuroendocrine tumors (NET). ASCO Gastrointestinal Cancers Symposium 2010 [abstract]. Available at: http://www.asco.org/ASCOv2/Meetings/Abstracts? &vmview=abst_detail_view&confID=72&abstractID=1797. Accessed April 20, 2010.

33. Kulke MH, Lenz HJ, Meropol NJ, et al. Activity of sunitinib in patients with advanced neuroendocrine tumors. J Clin Oncol 2008;26(20):3403–10.

34. Venook AP, Ko AH, Tempero MA, et al. Phase II trial of FOLFOX plus bevacizu-mab in advanced, progressive neuroendocrine tumors [abstract]. J Clin Oncol 2008;26(15S):15545.

35. Kulke M, Chan JA, Meyerhardt JA, et al. Phase II study of 2-methoxyestradiol (2ME2) administered in combination with bevacizumab, in patients (Pts) with advanced carcinoid tumors. ASCO Gastrointestinal Cancers Symposium 2008 [abstract]. Available at: http://www.asco.org/ascov2/Meetings/Abstracts? &vmview=abst_detail_view&confID=53&abstractID=10528. Accessed April 20, 2010.

36. Kulke MH, Stuart K, Enzinger PC, et al. Phase II study of temozolomide and thalidomide in patients with metastatic neuroendocrine tumors. J Clin Oncol 2006;24(3):401–6.

37. Yao JC, Zhang YX, Rashid A, et al. Clinical and in vitro studies of imatinib in advanced carcinoid tumors. Clin Cancer Res 2007;13(1):234–40.

38. Gross DJ, Munter G, Bitan M, et al. Israel glivec in solid tumors study group. The role of imatinib mesylate (Glivec) for treatment of patients with malignant endo-crine tumors positive for c-kit or PDGF-R. Endocr Relat Cancer 2006;13(2): 535–40.

39. Kulke MH, Bergsland EK, Ryan DP, et al. Phase II study of recombinant human endostatin in patients with advanced neuroendocrine tumors. J Clin Oncol 2006;24(22):3555–61.

40. Anthony L, Chester M, Michael S, et al. Phase II open-label clinical trial of vatalanib (PTK/ZK) in patients with progressive neuroendocrine cancer [abstract]. J Clin Oncol 2008;26(Suppl 20):14624.

41. Sung MW, Kvols L, Wolin E, et al. PhaseII proof-of-concept study of atiprimod in patients with advanced low-to intermediate-grade neuroendocrine carcinoma [abstract]. J Clin Oncol 2008;26(Suppl 20):4611.

42. Hobday TJ, Holen K, Donehower R, et al. A phase II trial of gefitinib in patients (pts) with progressive metastatic neuroendocrine tumors (NET): a phase II consortium (P2C) study [abstract]. J Clin Oncol 2006;24(18S):4043.

43. Hobday TJ, Rubin J, Holen K, et al. MC044h, a phase II trial of sorafenib in patients (pts) with metastatic neuroendocrine tumors (NET): a phase II consortium (P2C) study [abstract]. J Clin Oncol 2007;25(18S):4504.

44. Kulke M, Blaszkowski LS, Zhu AX, et al. PhaseI/II study of everolimus (RAD001) in combination with temozolomide (TMZ) in patients (pts) with advanced pancreatic neuroendocrine tumors (NET). ASCO Gastrointestinal Cancers Symposium 2010 [abstract]. Available at: http://www.asco.org/ASCOv2/Meetings/Abstracts?&vmview=abst_detail_view&confID=72&abstractID=2350. Accessed April 20, 2010.

45. Yao JC, Phan A, Chang DZ, et al. Phase II study of RAD001 (everolimus) and depot octreotide (sandostatin LAR) in advanced low grade neuroendocrine carcinoma (LGNET) [abstract]. J Clin Oncol 2007;25(18S):4503.

46. Kvols L, Wiedenmann B, Oberg K, et al. Safety and efficacy of pasireotide (SOM230) in patients with metastatic carcinoid tumors refractory or resistant to octreotide LAR: results of a phase II study [abstract]. J Clin Oncol 2006;24(18S):4082.

47. Faiss S, Pape UF, Böhmig M, et al. International lanreotide and interferon alfa study group. Prospective, randomized, multicenter trial on the antiproliferative effect of lanreotide, interferon alfa, and their combination for therapy of metastatic neuroendocrine gastroenteropancreatic tumors–the international lanreotide and interferon alfa study group. J Clin Oncol 2003;21(14):2689–96.

48. Rinke A, Müller HH, Schade-Brittinger C, et al. Placebo-controlled, double-blind, prospective, randomized study on the effect of octreotide LAR in the control of tumor growth in patients with metastatic neuroendocrine midgut tumors: a report from the PROMID study group. J Clin Oncol 2009;27(28):4656–63.

49. Brizzi MP, Berruti A, Ferrero A, et al. Continuous 5-fluorouracil infusion plus long acting octreotide in advanced well-differentiated neuroendocrine carcinomas. A phase II trial of the piemonte oncology network. BMC Cancer 2009;9:388.

50. Kulke MH, Stuart K, Enzinger PC, et al. Phase II study of temozolomide and thalidomide in patients with metastatic neuroendocrine tumors. J Clin Oncol 2006;24(3):401–6.

Index

Endocrinol Metab Clin N Am 39 (2010) 853–878
doi:10.1016/S0889-8529(10)00083-6
0889-8529/10/$ – see front matter © 2010 Elsevier Inc. All rights reserved.

endo.theclinics.com

United States Postal Service

Statement of Ownership, Management, and Circulation
(All Periodicals Publications Except Requestor Publications)

1. Publication Title: Endocrinology and Metabolism Clinics of North America	2. Publication Number: 0 0 0 - 2 7 7 5	3. Filing Date: 9/15/10

4. Issue Frequency: Mar, Jun, Sep, Dec	5. Number of Issues Published Annually: 4	6. Annual Subscription Price: $271.00

7. Complete Mailing Address of Known Office of Publication (Not printer) (Street, city, county, state, and ZIP+4®)

Elsevier Inc.
360 Park Avenue South
New York, NY 10010-1710

Contact Person: Stephen Bushing
Telephone (Include area code): 215-239-3688

8. Complete Mailing Address of Headquarters or General Business Office of Publisher (Not printer)

Elsevier Inc., 360 Park Avenue South, New York, NY 10010-1710

9. Full Names and Complete Mailing Addresses of Publisher, Editor, and Managing Editor (Do not leave blank)

Publisher (Name and complete mailing address)

Kim Murphy, Elsevier, Inc., 1600 John F. Kennedy Blvd. Suite 1800, Philadelphia, PA 19103-2899

Editor (Name and complete mailing address)

Rachel Glover, Elsevier, Inc., 1600 John F. Kennedy Blvd. Suite 1800, Philadelphia, PA 19103-2899

Managing Editor (Name and complete mailing address)

Catherine Bewick, Elsevier, Inc., 1600 John F. Kennedy Blvd. Suite 1800, Philadelphia, PA 19103-2899

10. Owner (Do not leave blank. If the publication is owned by a corporation, give the name and address of the corporation immediately followed by the names and addresses of all stockholders owning or holding 1 percent or more of the total amount of stock. If not owned by a corporation, give the names and addresses of the individual owners. If owned by a partnership or other unincorporated firm, give its name and address as well as those of each individual owner. If the publication is published by a nonprofit organization, give its name and address.)

Full Name	Complete Mailing Address
Wholly owned subsidiary of	4520 East-West Highway
Reed/Elsevier, US holdings	Bethesda, MD 20814

11. Known Bondholders, Mortgagees, and Other Security Holders Owning or Holding 1 Percent or More of Total Amount of Bonds, Mortgages, or Other Securities. If none, check box. ☐ None

Full Name	Complete Mailing Address
N/A	

12. Tax Status (For completion by nonprofit organizations authorized to mail at nonprofit rates) (Check one)
The purpose, function, and nonprofit status of this organization and the exempt status for federal income tax purposes:
☐ Has Not Changed During Preceding 12 Months
☐ Has Changed During Preceding 12 Months (Publisher must submit explanation of change with this statement)

PS Form 3526, September 2007 (Page 1 of 3 (Instructions Page 3)) PSN 7530-01-000-9931 PRIVACY NOTICE: See our Privacy policy in www.usps.com

---

13. Publication Title: Endocrinology and Metabolism Clinics of North America		14. Issue Date for Circulation Data Below: September 2010	

15. Extent and Nature of Circulation		Average No. Copies Each Issue During Preceding 12 Months	No. Copies of Single Issue Published Nearest to Filing Date
a. Total Number of Copies (Net press run)		2122	2101
b. Paid Circulation (By Mail and Outside the Mail)	(1) Mailed Outside-County Paid Subscriptions Stated on PS Form 3541. (Include paid distribution above nominal rate, advertiser's proof copies, and exchange copies)	711	692
	(2) Mailed In-County Paid Subscriptions Stated on PS Form 3541 (Include paid distribution above nominal rate, advertiser's proof copies, and exchange copies)		
	(3) Paid Distribution Outside the Mails Including Sales Through Dealers and Carriers, Street Vendors, Counter Sales, and Other Paid Distribution Outside USPS®	582	640
	(4) Paid Distribution by Other Classes Mailed Through the USPS (e.g. First-Class Mail®)		
c. Total Paid Distribution (Sum of 15b (1), (2), (3), and (4))	▶	1293	1332
d. Free or Nominal Rate Distribution (By Mail and Outside the Mail)	(1) Free or Nominal Rate Outside-County Copies Included on PS Form 3541	72	74
	(2) Free or Nominal Rate In-County Copies Included on PS Form 3541		
	(3) Free or Nominal Rate Copies Mailed at Other Classes Through the USPS (e.g. First-Class Mail)		
	(4) Free or Nominal Rate Distribution Outside the Mail (Carriers or other means)		
e. Total Free or Nominal Rate Distribution (Sum of 15d (1), (2), (3) and (4))	▶	72	74
f. Total Distribution (Sum of 15c and 15e)	▶	1365	1406
g. Copies not Distributed (See instructions to publishers #4 (page 45))	▶	757	695
h. Total (Sum of 15f and g)	▶	2122	2101
i. Percent Paid (15c divided by 15f times 100)		94.73%	94.74%

16. Publication of Statement of Ownership

If the publication is a general publication, publication of this statement is required. Will be printed in the December 2010 issue of this publication. ☐ Publication not required

17. Signature and Title of Editor, Publisher, Business Manager, or Owner

[signature] Stephen R. Bushing – Fulfillment/Inventory Specialist

Date: September 15, 2010

I certify that all information furnished on this form is true and complete. I understand that anyone who furnishes false or misleading information on this form or who omits material or information requested on the form may be subject to criminal sanctions (including fines and imprisonment) and/or civil sanctions (including civil penalties).

PS Form 3526, September 2007 (Page 2 of 3)

Moving?

Make sure your subscription moves with you!

To notify us of your new address, find your **Clinics Account Number** (located on your mailing label above your name), and contact customer service at:

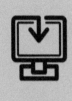

Email: journalscustomerservice-usa@elsevier.com

800-654-2452 (subscribers in the U.S. & Canada)
314-447-8871 (subscribers outside of the U.S. & Canada)

Fax number: 314-447-8029

Elsevier Health Sciences Division
Subscription Customer Service
3251 Riverport Lane
Maryland Heights, MO 63043

*To ensure uninterrupted delivery of your subscription, please notify us at least 4 weeks in advance of move.

Printed and bound by CPI Group (UK) Ltd, Croydon, CR0 4YY

03/10/2024

01040455-0017